A Survivor's Guide to
Study Skills and
Student Assessments

A Survivor's Guide to

For Churchill Livingstone:

Commissioning editor: Ellen Green
Project development editor: Valerie Bain
Project manager: Valerie Burgess
Design direction: Judith Wright
Design and electronic page make-up: Charles Simpson
Indexer: Tarrant Ranger Indexing Agency
Sales promotion executive: Hilary Brown

A Survivor's Guide to
Study Skills and Student Assessments
for health care students

Christopher J. Goodall

RGN DipN RNT
Visiting Lecturer, North Yorkshire College of Health Studies, York, UK

Illustrations by Lee Smith

CHURCHILL LIVINGSTONE
EDINBURGH LONDON MADRID MELBOURNE NEW YORK AND TOKYO 1995

CHURCHILL LIVINGSTONE
Medical Division of Pearson Professional Limited

Distributed in the United States of America by Churchill Livingstone
Inc., 650 Avenue of the Americas, New York, N.Y. 10011, and by
associated companies, branches and representatives throughout the
world.

First published 1995

ISBN 0 443 052484

British Library of Cataloguing in Publication Data
A catalogue record for this book is available from the British Library.

Library of Congress Cataloging in Publication Data
A catalog record for this book is available from the Library of
Congress.

The
publisher's
policy is to use
**paper manufactured
from sustainable forests**

Printed in Singapore

Contents

Preface

Standards of professional practice for nurses, physiotherapists and occupational therapists are jealously guarded, both to protect the public against poor standards of care, and to enhance the reputation of the profession. One means of achieving high standards of practice within the health care professions is to establish assessments throughout courses leading to professional qualifications.

These assessments form a vital part of the entire learning process, in that they contribute to the student's awareness of how much progress has been made. Assessments exist for the student's benefit, as much as for the college's or the public's.

Courses in health care, together with their assessments, set practitioners apart from the general public. Perhaps it is the case that the public *expects* health care professionals to be set apart from them, so that a nurse is privy to more detailed health care knowledge than is, say, a plumber or an artist.

For example, what is it that differentiates the loving care given to a sick child by a paediatric nurse on a hospital ward, and that given by the child's parents? Perhaps one measure is that the parents' care, while loving, is unplanned (though not unskilled). A nurse's care for a child *is* planned, based on a thorough appraisal of the needs of both the child and his parents. It is the nurse's professional training that teaches her to assess, plan, deliver, and evaluate skilled and appropriate care. It is the nurse's professional qualification that declares to the public her ability to carry out those stages of caring. And it is the assessments within health care courses that contribute to the award of a professional qualification.

This book was born out of a *cri de cœur* from one of my students: 'They set us these essays and care studies,' he declared, 'but they don't tell us what it is that they *want*.' Such a sentiment took me aback initially. Having given students essay titles myself, or criteria for writing a care study, I had assumed that students were well enough accustomed to writing essays and other assessments from having survived over a decade of schooling. Not so, apparently.

Further investigation revealed a lack of detailed, basic guidance about assessments in nurse training, and a profound sense of insecurity among students faced with such assessments. Once asked, students raised all sorts of questions: How much detail should I provide? Do I need to include references (and how do I write them)? What is this strange beast known as the 'academic style'? What does 'discuss' mean, and how is it different from 'describe'?

Essays came to me for marking which demonstrated a complete lack of awareness about the purpose of paragraphs. Such essays read more like an excerpt from a James Joyce 'flow-of-consciousness' novel than a well-planned in-depth discussion. Reviews of the literature consisted of little more than a succession of names and dates. As always, the prospect of examinations seemed to affect some students greatly, giving rise to levels of anxiety which were deeply worrying.

My own initially vague ideas about a text on student assessment coincided with similar, though firmer, suggestions from Churchill Livingstone... and this book is the result. It is aimed principally at student nurses, since it is nurse education with which I am most familiar. I have, however, tried to make it relevant to students of physiotherapy and occupational therapy. Medical students may also find it helpful.

As always, I am conscious of the enthusiasm, support and kindness of the staff at Churchill Livingstone, and I thank them most sincerely. Individuals' names are listed elsewhere. I am likewise indebted to colleagues of the North Yorkshire College of Health Studies, especially to Ian Dyson and Heather Cahill. The latter read, and commented on, Chapter 10, which helped me greatly (though any faults lie squarely at my door). I particularly want to thank Karen Smith, senior librarian of the college, and all her staff, who have been most helpful, and ever patient with me. I am grateful to Christine A. Mayers, principal lecturer, and Elizabeth McKay, professional practice coordinator, from the University College of Ripon & York St John, for their advice about occupational therapy education. A number of students have assisted me, both by discussing ideas that have cropped up during the writing of this book, and by helping me (as a disabled person) with practical matters. In both regards, Jerome Whitfield deserves my especial thanks.

This book is dedicated to two former senior tutors of the college – Joe Appleton and Jim Giddings – both of whom are now, alas, retired. I owe them much.

York, 1995   C.J.G.

Introduction

Almost every career you might choose to follow – teacher, concert pianist, or accountant – will have assessments you must pass. Even being an author has its assessments: your ability to write clearly and succinctly, to complete your script on time, and whether the public actually wants to buy your book.

Nurses and other health care professionals have many assessments to pass during their training, and this is partly to protect the public. Your patients will, after all, want to know that you can take their blood pressures accurately, and that you know how to manipulate a knee or hip joint safely. Both of these examples are of practical skills, but you will appreciate there is much more to health care than this.

You must know, for example, how to communicate clearly with your patients and clients and with other members of the health care team, both orally and in writing. When you plan a patient transfer to another ward, for example, you should be able to write a clear and accurate summary of his condition and management, so that the new nurses will be able to take over his treatment. Have a look at the following imaginary patient transfer note:

■ *Mr Jones, 42, abdo pain. Admitted from home this a.m. Routine obs, urinalysis OK, for further tests. Keep on bed rest, restrict fluids, relatives have phoned.*

As the receiving nurse you may not be greatly enlightened by this note. For example, what are those 'routine obs' you are supposed to be doing, and for what 'further tests' should you be preparing Mr Jones? And you haven't been told anything about Mrs Jones, who, desperately anxious about her husband, has to stay at home with their young daughter.

Written assessments, such as essays and care studies, help you to demonstrate how clearly, succinctly and accurately you can express yourself. The skills you utilize in an essay are very much the same skills you would use in writing a transfer note or drawing up a care plan – or, eventually, writing your own research study.

Throughout this book you'll find examples like the one above, sometimes with the suggestion that you write an improved version, or that you discuss with your colleagues the issues raised. In this way, this book is partly an *interactive* one, not a textbook to be read straight through. You'll be asked to pause for thought, to give an opinion, to make choices. The style of the book is informal (without, I hope, being annoyingly chatty) as if I were present, talking to you directly. You can't answer me back, or tell me you think I'm wrong, but you can certainly look at the examples I provide and attempt the exercises.

Who am I?

I have been a nurse teacher for over 10 years, teaching in both a Common Foundation Programme (CFP) and an Adult Branch. I also lecture on disability issues to student occupational therapists. I mark exam papers, essays, and project work from students at all stages of their courses. I'm well aware that the knowledge base of new students, just entering their education programme, can differ widely. One student can have recently obtained a degree in social sciences or biology, while another might not have studied for a long time, and might have few academic qualifications.

I have written extensively in the nursing press and elsewhere, and I hope that my articles have always shown an empathy with the special needs of both student nurses and those qualified nurses working at the bedside. A short time ago I wrote a workbook called *Exploring Physiology* (also published by Churchill Livingstone) to help students with their studies of human physiology. My aim with that book was to bring students with widely differing knowledge of physiology together to a common level of understanding.

The same applies to this present text. Students have different levels of confidence regarding studying for and passing assessments. Some will have got to grips with the process of assessment, having sailed through school and, perhaps, college and university without too much trouble. Others will be far less self-confident.

It is well known that individual students also have differing preferred methods of study. One of my aims in writing this guide to assessment is to help you discover which approach to studying is best for you.

Who are you?

You may have come into nursing, physiotherapy or occupational therapy straight from school. You might be a mature student, perhaps with a family of your own, who has entered one of the health care professions after several jobs or years spent raising children. If the latter, it is often the case that you're especially worried about getting into the swing of studying again after an absence from the classroom of 10 years or more. But be reassured. It is my experience that such students are highly motivated to study, and that their individual life experience helps them cope with most, if not all, of the assessments thrown at them.

You may feel you can deal with exams – after all, you might have just passed A levels or some other examinations. Others, however, sometimes feel ill with worry about approaching exams. This book aims to help you, both with your revision and with your psychological approach to exams.

Other students feel anxious about long project work, especially if they have to present their projects to an audience. Again, this book will help you.

About this book

This book is concerned mostly with written assessments – examinations, projects, and care studies – although the final chapter is about practical assessments. Many of the basic writing skills covered in the opening chapters will be applicable to most forms of written assessment, but there are some individual differences. It is my experience, for example, that students find writing a literature review very difficult, their efforts consisting of little more than a list of names and dates. Others are so awed by the word 'research' that they feel they can never subject someone else's research study to their own criticism. This book doesn't go into detail about the research process, or how to write your own research study – there are other books for that – but it sets out to give you the self-confidence to read a study carefully and critically.

Again in my experience, exam questions cause great problems for students, many of whom come to grief not because they don't know the information required, but because they have simply failed to answer the question as it is set. In this book I look at the difference between the common exam instructions 'describe' and 'discuss'. I look at the use of client or patient profiles within exam questions and show you how to spot important clues (rather like spotting the clues in a crime novel). That popular exam instruction, 'Using a problem-solving approach . . .' is also discussed. Students have failed such questions not because they didn't know the appropriate care, but because they didn't problem-solve in their answers.

This book is relatively brief. After all, in your health care course you'll have plenty of set texts to read – physiology, social policy and so on – besides this one. It will probably be most useful at the beginning of your course, but its contents may well stand revisiting as your studies progress (perhaps when a different form of assessment comes up). I hope, through its style and content, you will come to regard it – and its author – as a personal helpmate, one that will accompany you, and give you a word of encouragement, whenever you need it.

I dislike using the somewhat clumsy 'he or she' to deal with the problem of gender. Even more do I dislike the use of 's/he' which I find jars visually on the page. Consequently, I have decided to use the male pronoun in one paragraph, where appropriate, and the female pronoun in another. I have not attempted to alternate strictly between the two, nor – heaven forbid – to balance the number of *hes* and *shes* with the proportions of the sexes in nurse education, physiotherapy or occupational therapy. That would be beyond both my patience and my arithmetical skills.

Exercise is good for you

I said earlier that this book is, to some extent, interactive. Throughout it you'll find individual and group exercises in which you'll be asked, for example, to improve on passages provided to show poor examples. Such exercises are printed in special activity boxes, identified by their own icon.

These exercises, or activities, shouldn't be regarded as optional extras. This book's aim is to stimulate you to overcome possible difficulties *for yourself*, and one way of achieving this is to demonstrate, as you complete each exercise, that you are improving. 'Model answers' are not provided. Instead, I discuss possible approaches to the exercises given, discussion in which you are invited to join, perhaps with a group of fellow students.

Whenever I mark students' work, I feel somewhat overawed by the responsibility I've been given. To fail a project or an exam paper might be to end a youngster's career – and certainly to inflict great unhappiness on her. So I try and approach each paper or project in a positive frame of mind: Can I possibly *pass* this student? – rather than, Let's see how many *mistakes* I can find here.

The exercises in this book are offered in the same positive spirit. They are chances for you to try your best, to improve the quality of your work step by step, and even to shine! I will never know, of course, how well you do in each exercise (unless you write and tell me) but *you* will. *You* will see yourself growing more confident as your abilities increase, and this self-confidence can then be applied to your studies in nursing, physiotherapy or occupational therapy.

The improvement that you see in yourself, as you work your way through the exercises in this book, is yours – not mine, not this book's, but yours. You will become more self-critical, able to judge what is good in your own work, and what is less than good. You will know when to be satisfied with your work, and when not to be. This is a fine characteristic to take with you into your health care course.

Writing for publication

As well as activity boxes, this book includes boxes devoted to writing for publication, again with their own identifying icon. What is the link between written assessments and writing for publication? Such a link occurred to me while teaching in college. Within the same week I had to give a group of nurse finalists advice about writing exam answers, followed a little time later by a session on writing for publication to another student group.

It seemed to me that there were distinct similarities between submitting a soundly planned, neatly laid out typescript for, say, *Nursing Times,* and completing well-planned and presented answers to an exam. To give just one example: the initial impression made by both typescript and exam answer is highly important. The editor is pleased with what she finds, as is the marker, and both go on to consider the submitted piece of work in a positive frame of mind.

Further links should occur to you as you read each box. Alternatively, you may choose to ignore them if you have, at present, no interest in publishing. Incidentally, I should point out that the world of publishing is now immensely competitive. If you submit an article which is eventually rejected, you have no cause to believe your writing skills are inadequate. Journals such as *Nursing Times* and *Nursing Standard* receive over 50 unsolicited typescripts each week, from which only one or two may be chosen. Even established authors have their work rejected from time to time – as I well know.

This book contains a few further boxes devoted to writing technology, again identified by their own icon. Many students are nowadays well acquainted with computers and word processors, but for those who are not these boxes provide the bare minumum of information about the advantages (and drawbacks) of using today's writing and information machines. You *don't* have to own a word processor to be a good student, or even a good author. A crime writer friend of mine has published 26 books so far, each one written in longhand initially, then typed during the redrafting process. She has no intention of mastering the new technology, claiming that it makes for a careless writer. I must admit that, after using a word processor for about 5 years, I wouldn't be without it.

An additional feature of the book is the occasional appearance of margin tips, enclosed in their own 'bubbles'. These consist of summaries of the main text rather than additional points, and so may help you to skim through certain passages of the book until you arrive at the place you want. Look on them as 'helpful hints'.

So that you may personalize your copy of this book, blank pages have sometimes been left for your own comments and notes. These notes might, for example, refer to certain important assessment requirements of your own college, or timetables for study.

Notes

Notes

1

The assessment process

Key topics

- ■ **The purpose of assessment**
- ■ **How each individual assignment fits in the overall assessment strategy**

Introduction – the assessment process

Standing on a beach looking out to sea, you may not at first notice whether the tide is coming in or going out. All you can see is a succession of waves of varying sizes and ferocity coming towards you. It is only after the passage of time that you notice the tide is coming in, forcing you to move further up the beach.

So it is with the assessment process. On your health care course, you may at first see just a series of assessments heading towards you – relatively small assessments such as quizzes held in class, and much more forbidding assessments like a project or a 3-hour exam. Only after some time does the student notice that there is a direction, an overall strategy, to the assessments she tackles. In other words, there is an *assessment process* which moves each student in the direction of personal and professional development (Fig. 1.1).

It is likely that today's students are more aware of this process than I was during my general nurse training, through the provision of student handbooks by colleges, and the appointment of student members to curriculum development committees. Assessment is not a dark secret, brewed up behind locked doors by the assessment 'experts' (i.e. the teachers and managers). The assessment process for each college is something which is shared with the whole student body of that college. Students

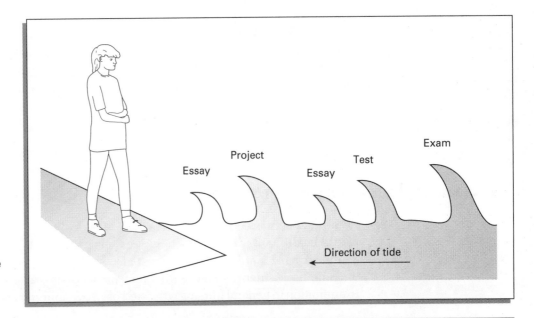

Figure 1.1
The student, at first unaware of the direction of the tide, sees just a succession of tests and exams heading towards her.

will want to know exactly what is expected of them, and to observe their own professional growth as much as will the teachers.

There is a logical movement throughout the process. Thus Test 2 builds on the achievements of Test 1 in terms of scope of knowledge and depth of understanding. The second test would be illogical without the initial stepping stone of the first test.

It is the same with the achievements gained from clinical placements on wards or fieldwork in the community. Colleges stipulate the achievements that are to be expected from a student's first placement, which will be different, in kind and in depth, to those gained in the second placement. Clinical placement mentors and assessors are well aware of these different levels of achievement; indeed, they may have played an important part in drawing up the clinical placement assessement strategy.

Here is an example of such a sequence.

> As a student nurse, physiotherapist or occupational therapist on your third clinical placement, you are asked to assess a new patient. During earlier placements you will have observed your mentor admitting and assessing patients in hospital. You will have noted the documentation used, and the way your mentor (an experienced practitioner) has adapted it to the individual needs of the patient. Perhaps on your second placement you will have led an admission procedure with your mentor in close attendance, to give advice when necessary. Now you are ready to go solo.

> Your initial contact with your patient – greeting her, observing her facial expression, listening to her first few replies to your questions – leads you to suspect that she is a little unsure about the reasons for her admission. Realizing this, you adapt the admission procedure by bringing forward questions about the patient's understanding of her condition. You feel it is important to be clear about this early on, rather than plough on through the documentation, asking the set questions exactly as they're written.

> Discussing this afterwards with your mentor, she congratulates you on having the courage – and the basic understanding of the principles of patient assessment – to carry out this adjustment. Without those few earlier experiences when you observed a patient being admitted to the ward, you might not have seen the necessity for doing this, and an important opportunity for building a relationship with your patient could have been lost.

Assessments, whether they are written or practical, consist of more than a series of tasks to be ticked off as they're carried out. Each assessment within the overall assessment strategy takes over the 'learning baton' from its predecessor, and develops it so that it is ready to be handed over to the next (Fig. 1.2).

Those who devise health care courses know very well that an assessment cannot 'double back' on the overall direction taken by the assessment process. The runner cannot turn round and head back the way she came, carrying the learning baton with her. Each assessment must constitute a lap in the overall race, and the race is towards the goal of personal and professional growth (a goal which, you'll realize, is never fully achieved).

> Don't confuse patient assessment with your own assessment as a student.

The role of feedback in the assessment process

Without effective feedback from teachers at every step of the assessment process, it would be difficult for students to judge their progress. We all feel better for praise, and work harder after it, but we must also know where we've gone wrong.

Some assessments carry with them no feedback at all. My own State Final Examination in general nursing consisted of two 3-hour papers, after which I received

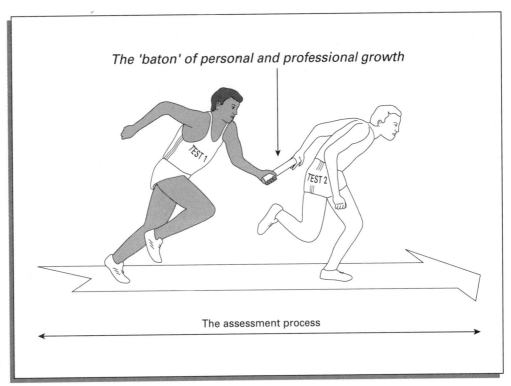

The 'baton' of personal and professional growth

The assessment process

Figure 1.2
Assessments build on the personal
and professional growth demonstrated
in earlier assessments.

notification that I had passed. To this day I have no idea whether I produced the best papers the examiners had ever seen, or whether I only just managed to scrape by. Because I'd passed, this didn't bother me – but what about those students who had failed? The examiners offered them no individual help, no feedback on their efforts, beyond publishing general comments on the overall standard of the answers.

It must have been difficult, too, for tutors of those students. What advice could they offer their students for further revision and exam practice if there was no individual feedback?

In my own college of health studies, students who fail module exams, projects or care studies, are given written comments by the examiners so that revision towards resubmission can be better directed. Even if the student's first attempt at the college's final exam ends in failure, examiners' comments are provided – a much more responsible attitude, in my view, to both assessment and the student.

Students on health care courses should be aware that some assessments are *formative* while others primarily are *summative*. An examination at the end of a course, for which there is the award of a pass or fail grade, is an example of a summative assessment. Such assessments usually mark the final point or an important part of a course. (For example, a nurse's common foundation programme and branch programme might each end with a summative assessment in the form of an exam.)

Formative assessments are those which occur *en route*, and for which feedback is all important. These assessments play a vital role in the student's awareness of her personal and professional development. For this to be the case, a marker's comments at the bottom of an essay are far more valuable than simply a score. The benefit of such comments depends on their clarity, accuracy and detail. 'A good attempt, though more detail is required in places' is, I would suggest, of little use to the student.

In practice, assessments in health care courses are more often a mixture of formative and summative. A module examination can mark an important course milestone, one that must be passed before the student can go on to the next; but it will also provide useful feedback in the form of written comments from the marker(s).

The student should guard against viewing formative assessments as less important than summative. It is as important to discover one's personal and professional growth (or lack of it) from a formatively assessed essay, as it is to pass a summatively assessed project or exam.

In the next chapter I shall be looking at individuals' preferences for study methods.

2 Individual approaches to study

Key topics

■ **Basic study skills such as:**
  —managing your study time
  —taking notes
  —assembling your data

In a health care course of approximately 3 years, each student must not only overcome each assessment that comes her way but, in so doing, must devise her own individual style of studying.

Just as a learner driver learns not only about driving a car or motorcycle, but also about how to pass the test, so the health care student has to come to grips with the problem of passing assessments as well as the art and science of caring for people.

In order to survive the assessments that come your way throughout your course, and in order to progress in the right direction along the assessment process of your college, you need to identify those strategies of studying that suit you. This chapter identifies some of these strategies, but only you can decide which suit you best.

Facilities for study

You may live in a hospital residence or your own home. You may have noisy neighbours or considerate ones. You may live on your own or, as with many mature students, with your family. If the latter, it is often difficult to balance your needs for studying and the needs of your partner and/or children.

My preference is for studying in solitude and complete silence. I find I cannot concentrate with background music playing – to me, music is for listening to, not something to keep me company. Nevertheless, others find that silence unnerves them, and they cannot work in the isolation which silence suggests. Therefore they switch on the radio in order to provide the impression of company.

Whatever your final choice of study facilities, there should be adequate overhead lighting to avoid straining your eyes. Your desk or table should have enough space for notes, typewriter or word processor, textbooks, and dictionary. Everything you need, in short, should be to hand.

It is perhaps worthwhile setting yourself the first few months of your course to discover what type of study conditions best suits you. You could try working in the college library for a week, and then in your own room, on your own and then with the company of your fellow students, in silence and with background music.

Some students may not have any choice. For them, study must proceed as best it can against the hubbub of family distractions. If it is possible, such a student should attempt to fix up a 'study space' which is hers alone, somewhere where books and notes can be left undisturbed. Students could attempt to make contracts with other family members for periods of undisturbed (relative) peace. Partners may even be persuaded to cook meals once in a while, or change the nappy of a crying baby. I do

> If working at home, establish a study area that is yours alone.

realize, however, that despite everyone's best efforts, being a parent will take precedence over an essay that urgently needs completing. There is no doubt that mature students with families have greater hurdles to leap than those on their own. Consequently, I know that the advice that follows could well be greeted by some mature students with hollow laughter.

Managing your time

Once a written assessment has been set, you should draw up a timetable for both its preparation and completion. Only you will know how fast you can work, or whether or not you work best under pressure. (Most of us do, incidentally, but that's no excuse for leaving things till the last minute.)

Allow yourself time for looking through libraries, for sending away for articles not immediately available, and for discussing the assignment with your colleagues. Allow time for the topic simply to 'brew' inside your head.

Make use of your personal organizer to establish specific study tasks for certain days, or you can use a diary that's big enough to take detailed entries for each day.

Your timetable might include the following headings:

- background reading
- selection of references
- making notes
- planning
- seek tutor's advice
- first draft
- seek tutor's advice
- second draft. This might be your final draft, depending on your tutor.

Do not expect to produce a brilliant 'final draft' at the first attempt. Writing successive drafts is a hard slog, made somewhat easier by the use of a word processor.

WORD PROCESSORS

These machines are excellent aids to a student or writer, but they aren't absolutely necessary. If you are contemplating buying a word processor, do seek the advice of someone who has one or who is well used to them. You can easily spend many hundreds of pounds on a machine which turns out not to be right for you.

All you have to do, after drawing up your timetable, is to *stick to it*. Remember there will be other areas of your health care course where work may be set, quite apart from the assignment you're currently planning to write. Allow time for such unpleasant additions to your workload, but also allow yourself time for relaxation.

How long should you work at a stretch? Only you can know this. Only you can judge that moment where, as the print in front of your tired eyes begins to swim, you know there is no point in going on. I would guess that 2 hours is many people's limit for working before having a break. Your limit might be just 1 hour.

You might consider working out a system of rewards for completing each 'block' of work, however long it is for you. For example, as I am very fond of coffee, I usually promise myself: work for the next $1\frac{1}{2}$ hours, *then* make myself a cup of coffee. This way, I'm rewarding myself for achieving my set block of study. The trouble with, by contrast, taking a cup of coffee to my desk and drinking it as I work, is that the coffee drinking takes over from the studying I'm supposed to be doing. I drink and daydream, rewarding myself (with the coffee) for *not* working effectively.

Your particular choice of reward might be a hot bath, or a 3-mile run, or listening to a record. If you live in hospital residences with other members of your course, you can establish joint rewards with your friends. Make a pact: Let's all meet in the Common Room in 2 hours' time for coffee and a chat. Here the reward is coffee and socialization. This may prove more practical than trying to work together in a group. I've never found studying with others helpful, but you will have to decide that for yourself.

Don't kid yourself

I am a great believer in my ability to kid myself. After sitting at my desk for some time, and beginning to feel like *another* cup of coffee, I'll tell myself: You deserve a break; you must have been studying for *hours*. A glance at my watch tells me that, sadly, I've put in only 45 minutes.

Studying for exams some years ago, I used a kitchen timer and some graph paper as a means of checking on my study time. The timer was set as I began to study, so that after an hour it rang and I knew how long I'd been working. I drew up a 'Study Chart' on the graph paper so that each hour of studying – each genuine, timed hour – meant a shaded square. Each week, I built up a column of shaded squares, as in Figure 2.1, and this became another reward – seeing how high I could get each week's column. I was elated when one week's score exeeded the previous week's, dejected when it was less.

You might try a similar system for yourself, but beware of believing what you want to believe – that you've put in hours and hours of study. It might be true, but all too often it isn't.

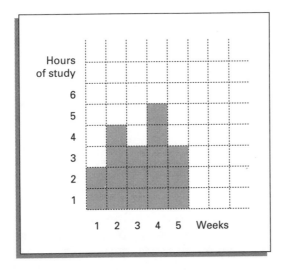

Figure 2.1
Recording study time in 1-hour 'blocks'.

Lectures and literature: summarizing and taking notes

It is likely that in your health care course you will be given both lectures and reading lists. Sometimes lectures will be followed by discussions among small groups of students guided by a teacher. These are very useful, because they help to develop ideas presented in lectures, and to sort out any misunderstandings students may have. Never be too shy to join in such discussions, even though you feel as if you're the dimmest member. You probably aren't. That all too simple question you're dying to ask, but daren't because it will make you look foolish, is the very question the other students are hoping someone else will ask.

Students have, somewhat naturally, differing opinions about the value of lectures. They are often presented to large groups of students, and there is usually far less opportunity to ask questions than in seminars. Sometimes it's difficult to hear a speaker in a large room, or to see his overhead projector (OHP) diagrams. (See Chapter 9 for advice on using OHPs effectively.) Students sometimes feel they can derive more useful information from reading textbooks than from listening to lectures. When reading, they can arrange for breaks that suit their own learning pace. In lectures this isn't possible.

One advantage of lectures over books, however, is that the information given can be much more up to date. As an author, I well know the frustrating delay between writing something and its appearing in print, the delay being longer for books than for articles. So a lecture can provide new ideas that the teacher is currently working on. For example, I give my present students a lecture on models of disability, at the end of which I provide a reading list of references, but I am presently developing a model of disability about which I haven't yet written. In my lecture I can describe this model to students and even, from their reactions to it, adjust it, which benefits both students and myself.

Your notes taken during a lecture should complement those you make when reading. In a lecture, I can direct students to those references I feel are most useful, or most readable. 'Try Jones first,' I can advise, 'but leave Smith alone until you're sure you can understand what Jones has to say.' Books and articles can, however, provide much more information than a lecture lasting 1 hour. With written material, you can go back and reread something you didn't understand the first time. It is likely, therefore, that the bulk of your notes will be derived from the literature.

The golden rule is *always to take notes when you read*. This will at first appear to slow your studying down. It is much quicker to get through a long list of references simply by reading them without taking any notes. You know, however, that you will never remember all the important facts and arguments (unless you're blessed with a photographic memory) so notetaking is an essential part of your reading.

> Always make notes when you read recommended texts – it helps you organize your knowledge.

ACTIVITY

Take a short time to study Figures 2.2 and 2.3. Whatever the merits of the information contained there, see if you can understand their logic. The diagrams are based on the same facts, so it should be easy to move from one system to the other. Which do you think suits you better? Could you improve on either figure?

Try this exercise with a group of your colleagues. Draw up for yourselves a short list of further information that might be added to the figures provided. For example, you could add 'Elderly people' and 'The chronically ill' as major categories of people affected by poverty; and as subheadings you could add 'Effects on housing' to match the 'Effects on diet' already there. Think of some more additions to my suggestions, then discuss how you would incorporate these in both the subheading and the flow diagram formats. What comments do you have about either?

Another useful exercise would be to set yourselves the task of producing notes from an article chosen by your group, or suggested by your teacher. Make it a fairly brief, factual one that is related to your course. Set yourselves a specific time in which to read the article and make your notes. This in itself will be a learning experience, but even more so will be the discussion and comparison of your notes when members of the group meet afterwards.

Are there important differences between the notes written by your colleagues? Are some notes considerably more detailed than others? If so, is this to their benefit or not? Be prepared to justify the way in which you've made your own notes.

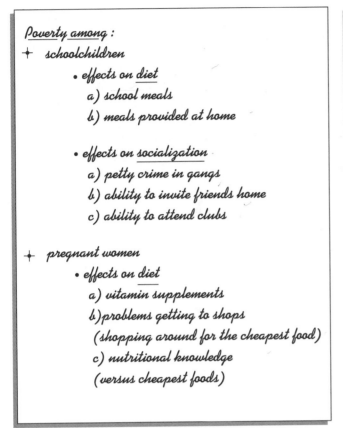

Figure 2.2
Making notes, using headings and subheadings.

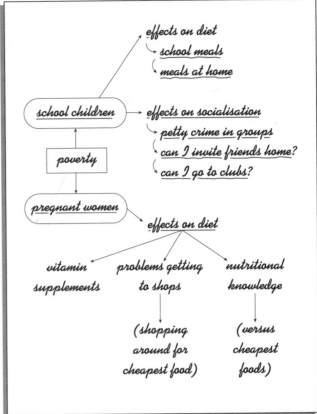

Figure 2.3
Making notes, using a 'flow diagram'.

Ogier
p.47

The way you make notes is obviously very personal. You may find it useful to incorporate headings and subheadings so as to organize the information you're collecting. Others will use 'flow diagrams'. These two techniques are illustrated in Figures 2.2 and 2.3, utilizing the same information.

Each system has its problems. Using 'flow diagrams' as in Figure 2.3, I've sometimes run off the edge of the paper because more additional facts have come along than I anticipated. With headings and subheadings, however, I find it easier to grasp an overall structure for the subject being studied.

Your skills in making notes, whether from lectures or the literature, will centre on your ability to *summarize*. There is little point in your notes consisting of a word-for-word repetition of what appears in the book in front of you. You must be able to pick out the important facts and the most relevant supporting detail, and then record them in such a way that it will make sense to you when you come to read your notes, perhaps several months afterwards.

It may be that an author has expressed a particularly important point in an especially pithy way, one that you feel you can't compress or improve on. In such a case, it may be worth quoting the author directly. You must, however, acknowledge the quotation by providing an exact reference (see Ch. 7). Also, don't make such quotations too long. It's your work, not the author's.

The opening few weeks of your course may provide you with opportunities to practise notetaking which is, after all, a skill that mentally stretches most people. Alternatively, or additionally, you can make opportunities to practise in small groups as I suggested earlier. The key is to pick out the most important facets of the lecture or article and to record them clearly. This has to be done in a very limited time if you are taking notes from a lecture.

With the wide provision of photocopiers in colleges, you may feel tempted to take a copy of a useful article you find. There is an understandable feeling of reassurance when the copy is safely installed in your notes folder. However, photocopying does not fix the essential details of the article in your mind! Some cynical teachers may believe that students, once they've copied an article, never actually get round to reading it.

Please understand that photocopying does not replace the need to take careful notes. In fact, by your refusal to take a copy and your insistence on making notes instead, you are not only saving trees and college bills, you are participating far more robustly, honestly and effectively in the learning process.

Assembling your information

Let me assume you have now carried out the reading suggested by your assignment title, and have written notes. While you've been reading around the subject, ideas may have suggested themselves to you about how the essay might be tackled. Now you need to arrange your notes so that they aid your understanding of the set subject.

It's as if your information is being condensed stage by stage. From, say, 100 pages of the literature, you've created 12 pages of notes, but even this is too much to give you an overview.

One suggestion is to use either small pieces of paper or record cards on which to write information under important headings, one card per heading. I use record cards that are readily available at stationers, the best size for me being 152 by 101 mm (6 in x 4 in).

Suppose I'm set an essay on poverty among children and its effect on their health. In my reading I've made notes on the following subjects:

- the prevalence of poverty among schoolchildren from 1979 to 1991
- changes in welfare benefits from 1970 to 1991
- the alleged widening of the gap between rich and poor from 1979
- rising rates of juvenile crime since 1985
- smoking among schoolchildren in the 1980s
- alcohol consumption among teenagers
- relative cheapness of alcohol in 1990 compared with 1970.

All this information is spread across 12 pages of notes. I've also acquired three newspaper reports – I'm beginning to panic. How can I get this into order so that it makes sense? This is where my cards can help. What I want is information 'at a glance'. To achieve this, I write short headings on my cards, below which I can write the most important facts together with their references. For example, the first three subjects listed above could be reduced to the following headings on their record cards:

- schoolchild poverty, '79–'91
- benefits changes, '70–'91
- rich–poor gap from '79.

Figure 2.4 shows an example of one of those record cards. Look at it, not to judge the information it contains, but to see how it's expressed concisely yet with relevant references. This card will lead me to precisely the correct article or page of my notes.

The next stage in the process of information handling is to 'shuffle the pack' (Fig. 2.5). What I now do is to 'shape' my essay by arranging and rearranging my record cards with their brief pieces of information. Should 'Rich–poor gap' come before or after 'Benefits changes'? Would 'Poverty, definition' make a sensible introduction to

BENEFITS CHANGES, '70-'91

- OPCS surveys begun '84 ⎫
      finished '89   ⎬ Hillyard 1992
- 'The way ahead' Jan '90 ⎭ pp. 127-131
- Creation of dependency (see notes p.5)
- Lack of knowledge re benefits (p.7) & poor take up (p.9)
- Social fund 1988
- Freezing child benefit (p.11)
- discretionary loans (pp.3-4)
- Government aim to better 'target' benefits (p.6) (Johnson 1991, P.11)

Figure 2.4
Record cards – brief headings plus subheadings and references.

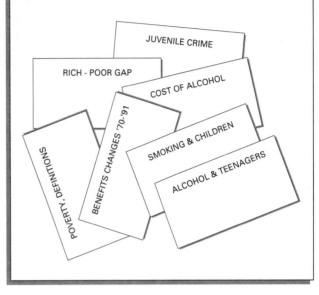

Figure 2.5
Planning your essay – 'shuffling the pack'.

the essay? Obviously, 'Alcohol & teenagers' should come next to 'Cost of alcohol' – but in which order?

You see the beauty of having snippets of important information arranged on these cards? In this way you have 'data at a glance', information which is far more easily handled than rustling desperately through pages and pages of notes and articles. There's no point in gathering information if you can't retrieve it in order to make use of it. Having a vague feeling that you've 'got something somewhere on child poverty' is not much use to you. Knowing where you can put your hands on it exactly, is the key to handling information.

It is quite possible to build your information into a logical structure, using record cards or slips of paper, before you begin to write your assignment. This is preferable to hoping for a structure to emerge as you write. Structure tends not to flow naturally off the nib of your pen, yet it is what gives an assignment a satisfying and convincing shape.

> Store the information you gain from reading so that you can easily retrieve it when needed.

Finally – look after yourself

At this point it is well worth mentioning the importance of taking care of your own health. Studying is exhausting as well as exciting. When you're making notes from a collection of articles you've discovered, there is the temptation to say 'Just one more page, *then* I'll stop.' One more becomes another one, then another, and so on. No one else is going to force you to stop and take a break – only you can.

I don't believe you study effectively on a diet of black coffee, cigarettes and late nights. Rest and relaxation, fresh air, exercise, and good nutrition play their part in the process of learning. Look after your mind and your career by looking after yourself.

One advantage of studying in a small group is that fellow students are well placed to notice signs of strain in a colleague. Periods of socialization are appropriate for sharing any concerns about your progress with your friends. They are also useful for listening to others' concerns. Sometimes people choose inappropriate means of reducing stress, such as cigarettes and alcohol. Drinking a can of beer with your group at the end of a study evening can be relaxing, but sometimes over-reliance develops. The person concerned may not be aware of this happening, but his friends are well placed to notice the danger signs. Make your group a sort of 'therapeutic community': a community that, learning how to care for others, also cares for its own members.

3

Essential preparation for written assessments

Key topics

- ■ The significance of written assessments within the assessement process
- ■ Important information about your college's assessment strategy, as it concerns your written assignment

Introduction – why do we need written assessments?

One of the first essays I wrote in the Introductory Course of my general nurse training was entitled, 'How to make a bed'. This followed a week's practice making empty beds in our Practical Room. Even in those days of meek student compliance to our elders and betters, all of us afterwards agreed that it was a ridiculous subject for an essay.

What did our teachers hope to gain from reading our essays? Presumably, whether or not we knew how to make a bed. They would also have learned whether we could write neatly, spell and punctuate correctly, and order our thoughts logically. They would have learned whether we could follow simple assessment instructions, such as including a margin, or writing on both sides of the page, or keeping to the set word limit. So that particular essay was perhaps not such a waste of time as we thought – but I am sure you will be able to think immediately of a much better assessment technique for testing students' bedmaking skills.

Initially it may seem strange that training for practical careers such as nursing should be tested by means of written assessments, including exams. In fact, the practical skills of nursing, physiotherapy and occupational therapy are rigorously tested, usually by the assessors and mentors in the areas where you gain practical experience. They will observe your dexterity, your manner in dealing with a client's problems, your safety in, say, administering medicines. But there is much more to health care professional practice than the routine performance of practical jobs.

Writing an essay or project will show your ability to address a particular problem – the topic set by your teacher. It will demonstrate your ability to organize yourself and your time so that you pay the task of planning and writing your assignment the attention it deserves.

To complete a written assignment well is to prove to yourself, as well as your marker, that you can:

- ● plan your time
- ● discover and read relevant texts
- ● assimilate from those texts important information
- ● form that information into a logical sequence
- ● address your mind to the data you've collected and arranged so that you come to a logical conclusion about it
- ● reproduce your discussion, clearly, in written form, within the required time and word limit.

I suspect that if you can achieve all these, you will be well pleased with yourself. Indeed, the act of writing an assignment (and especially writing the very last full stop) is particularly satisfying. It is even more satisfying should the assignment topic be one that initially didn't appeal to you. It might have bored you, or frightened you – yet you overcame your feelings and delivered your study or essay on time. Writing is, believe me, a pleasure as well as a pain.

What you need to know before you start work

The title

Make sure you are clear about the exact title set by your tutor. Every word should be regarded as being significant. Are there certain words you don't fully understand? For example:

■ *Discuss the effects of poverty on infant morbidity and mortality.*

Whatever the merits or otherwise of this essay topic, there are at least three words you need to be sure about before even doing the preparatory reading. What, for example, do the terms 'morbidity' and 'mortality' mean? They sound somewhat similar, but are they? Also, how is the word 'infant' defined? Does it simply mean a very young child, or is there a specific age range?

You may also wonder about that important term 'poverty' which, after all, is going to be central to your discussion. Rather like 'infant', is this a vague term meaning 'not very well off', or is there a precise definition? If so, where is this definition to be found: in an English dictionary or in one of your set texts on, say, social policy? (In other words, does it have a specialized meaning within the context of your health care course?)

Words are important. They can sometimes mean different things in different settings, but often they have exact definitions. Don't use words carelessly. It is a good habit, when you read, to have a dictionary by you, and to note those words whose meaning you don't know.

If you have any doubts about an essay title you've been set, seek the guidance of your tutors.

You should be sure whether or not you are being offered a choice of essay or project subject. The key is to read the instructions at the head of the paper giving the assignment topic(s). Are there choices *hidden* within an assignment? For example, the question given earlier might have been written thus:

■ *Discuss the effects of poverty on infant morbidity or mortality.*

Can you see the difference? Just one word has been changed, and so has the essay. To be fair, most choices would have been shown more clearly, like this:

■ *Discuss the effects of poverty on* either *infant morbidity* or *infant mortality.*

Even so, as many experienced markers will tell you, it is often the case that a few students' essays on this subject would embrace both morbidity and mortality, failing to notice the choice within the essay title.

The word count

The instructions for your assignment will tell you of how many words it should consist. A typical word count for an essay on a given topic might be 3000. Before you gasp with horror at such a number, be assured that, more often than not, you will have more problems *reducing* your essay to the required length than reaching it.

Please do note the word count. Bear it in mind as you begin to write your assignment, having first assembled the necessary relevant information. Your word count may be expressed as a range: for example, 2500 to 3500 words. If so, you should certainly ensure your assignment falls between the two numbers. If the word count is a single number, you and your colleagues will need to clarify from your teacher how far away from the provided count you may safely stray. (No teacher is going to expect you to meet the word count precisely.) For example, with a required word count of 3000, an essay of 2750 or 3100 words could well be acceptable, whereas one of 5500 would not.

If you use a word processor, it is likely that it will incorporate a word count facility. For those who still rely on ballpoint, fountain pen or quill, you will need to gain some idea of what the required word count looks like.

 ACTIVITY

How many words are there on one full A4 page in your handwriting? Work out first an average number of words per line. Count up the words on, say, five complete lines of a piece of your handwritten work. The score may be something like 55 words on five lines. Divide the total (55) with the number of lines (5) and you reach an average word score per line. Now count the number of lines per page (it may be something like 32 lines) and multiply this by the average line word count. What answer have you arrived at, using the figures I've provided? Indented lines, or lines omitted, will of course affect the word count of a page.

If you intend to 'double space' a handwritten essay – that is, use alternate lines– this will halve your word count per page.

Depending on the size and sprawl of your handwriting, you'll probably arrive at a word count per single-spaced A4 page of approximately 330. If you double space, your word count per page will be something like 170.

Hand-in date

You will be notified of the hand-in date at the same time as you are given the assignment's title and word count. Note it well. Write it in your diary, and perhaps write reminders 1 week and 2 weeks (and perhaps even more) before the date.

The problem is, of course, that if you are set a hand-in date 4 months ahead, it is all too easy to kid yourself that you have lots of time. You haven't. The time you've been set to complete your assignment will have been calculated to allow for reading, thinking, and planning, as well as writing. It is, I'm afraid, poor organization to leave everything till the last few days.

Most if not all colleges will have regulations covering the eventuality of a student falling ill and so not being able to meet a submission date. Usually, your course manager will grant an extension for the completion of an assignment if she believes there is good cause – such as ill health or a serious family problem. Having a hangover, not feeling like doing anything, or too many late-night parties, may not count as adequate causes for an extension.

Be aware, too, of your college's regulations concerning non-submission of a piece of work. In other words, you've failed both to hand an assignment in on time, and to seek an extension. Many colleges, in these circumstances, would award a Fail grade. This could have serious consequences for you continuing with your course.

Note also that hand-in dates sometimes stipulate a time of day as well as a date. For example, 'Essays must be handed in by 12 midday on Friday 28 January.' Usually colleges stipulate that it is the student's responsibilty to ensure her essay lands on the right desk at the right time. Excuses such as 'lost in the post', or 'given to a friend who forgot it', will tend not to be accepted.

Complying with the hand-in date demonstrates your ability to manage your time: both the time you devote to study and the time you set aside for recreation.

How the assignment is to be presented

You should read and follow instructions concerning the presentation of your work. These may include whether it must be typed, and whether illustrations are required. Some colleges ask for two copies of each piece, so as to help the moderation process.

By 'illustrations' I mean those which are relevant to the subject you are discussing. I have sometimes received projects written on pink paper and decorated with crayonned buttercups and daisies. You do not gain marks for pretty flowers. Illustrations should help to illuminate the text, and should have an explanatory caption. If there is more than one illustration, they should be numbered (Figure 1, Figure 2, and so on).

It is very important that you number your pages. Markers will find it impossible to supply a list of comments if they aren't able to refer to specific pages.

Follow instructions concerning margins. You may be asked for a $1^1/_2$ inch left hand margin (usually so that comments can be written there) or for margins all round the text. If you are fitting your pages into a binder, allow a really good left hand margin so that you don't lose some of your text in the binding. Experiment before you type out your fair copy.

WRITING FOR PUBLICATION

When submitting typescripts to professional journals for consideration, you will find that each journal has its own wishes concerning presentation of material. Often, a wide, all-round margin is stipulated, so that editors' and printers' comments can be added. Pages should only be typed or printed on one side. Many editors prefer that a typescript is held together with a paperclip, not a staple. This is so that printers can work on pages that are completely flat. It is important that your typescript contains your name and address, the article's title, and its length.

If you are using a word processor, do not 'justify' the right margin. It is easier for the printer to judge how many pages of print your article will take up when there is an unjustified right margin (even though it may look a bit ragged and untidy).

Just as you shouldn't exceed the word count for an essay you've been set, so you should keep to the restraints preferred by your chosen journal. An editor looking for a 1100 word article on physiotherapy in the elderly may consider a piece that's 1250 words long. A submission that is, say, 4500 words in length would probably not be given a second glance because it would entail far too much editorial time.

Pleasing a prospective editor is very like pleasing the marker of your assignment. Everything about your work – article or essay – should be designed to make her job easier.

Sometimes students use a folder for their essays whereby every page is slipped into a clear plastice sleeve. This is excellent for keeping their work clean, but the marker has to extricate each page on which comments have to be written – a time-consuming job which won't do anything to soothe his or her savage breast. Do everything you can, short of enclosing a £5 note, to make your marker's task easier.

Are references required?

In order to discuss the subject set for your assignment, you will need to read up on it and make notes. In today's diploma and degree level health care courses, it is more often than not a requirement that you should include references to the literature. How to set out references, and the different methods available, are subjects covered in Chapter 7. Here I'll simply say that the inclusion of references allows you to make assertions with safety.

For example, you are set an essay on 'Alcohol abuse among teenagers'. In the course of your essay, you feel justified in writing something like:

■ *Today's teenagers are far better acquainted with alcohol than those in the postwar years. Nowadays, it is much more likely for parents to face a drunken son or daughter returning home from a party.*

> Use references to the literature to back up statements you make in written assessments.

If you are a parent yourself, or indeed if you are still a teenager with first-hand experience of drunken parties, you might feel able to make such claims. But are you? Do you *really* know what alcohol consumption was like in the 1940s and 1950s, and what it is like across Britain today?

On the other hand, in your preparatory reading for this essay, you may have come across some research by Brown & Smith in 1991, which bears out exactly what you are claiming. This would therefore be an excellent reference to include in your essay.

Be sure that you know whether your college expects references to be included and which reference method is preferred (see Ch. 7). The instructions for your assignment might even mention that certain marks are awarded for the correct use of references, and you would be very wise to note this. Otherwise you could be throwing away 20% or 30% of the possible marks (see the next section). Incidentally, there is more to using references than dotting authors' names and dates throughout the text. Again, this is covered in Chapter 7.

How are the marks awarded?

One important part of the guidelines your college provides for the assignments it sets you, concerns the weighting of the marks awarded.

An essay might appear in two parts with, say, 30% of the marks awarded to Part A and 70% of the marks awarded to Part B. This weighting will tell you how much time and effort should be applied to each part; most often, though, this splitting of the marks occurs in examination questions.

Essays and longer projects more usually attract 100%, with no division of the set topic into parts. However, different weight may be awarded by the markers to different aspects of your answer. If this is the case, students should be clearly aware of the arrangement. Here is an example of such weighting:

Presentation (handwriting, grammar, spelling)	10%
Use of references to the literature	25%
How well the essay is organized and answers the question set	65%

You will notice that to forget all about including references to the literature in your answer, under the scheme above, is to reduce your maximum possible mark to 75%. To misread or misunderstand the question, however, invites disaster, since you will have thrown away 65 marks. It is certainly my experience, in marking both essays and exam answers, that more students fail through answering a different question from the one actually set, than from providing inaccurate information.

In this chapter I have shown how important it is for the student to read and note all the instructions provided for each assessment. Any point which seems the slightest bit obscure should be clarified with your teacher, before you spend time following your studies in the wrong direction.

Seeking your tutor's help

I would add one further factor that you need to be clear about from the outset: what level of tutorial help is available to you, and at what stage(s) it can be sought.

Sometimes, colleges stipulate exactly how and when tutors may help their students in the preparation of a piece of work. This is partly to ensure equal help for all students – it is then up to each student to seek that help. It is also, in part, designed to protect the teacher. There is the possibility that a teacher reads through his student's work in rough draft and (unwisely, as it turns out) declares that it is fine, and that it deserves to pass. When, following submission, the study earns a fail grade, the student feels naturally aggrieved.

To prevent this happening, a college may stipulate that tutors may see only a care study outline, or small sections of the study itself, prior to submission. I would suggest this is most likely to happen where care studies are marked not by students' own tutors but by a 'pool' of markers, sometimes even from a separate college site or campus.

I should add that all colleges make strenuous efforts to ensure that individual teachers mark consistently and to established criteria, so that a student's study would gain practically the same mark no matter which teacher marked it. The system of internal and external moderation helps to achieve this. Nevertheless, many students are aware of the rumour (rather than the fact) that Miss X is a much tougher marker than Dr Y. In fact such reputations are usually undeserved, as marking workshops attended by teachers will demonstrate.

Interestingly, in one of my positions as an external examiner, I noticed how many students hesitated to seek tutorial advice about their set essays. To them it seemed that this almost constituted cheating. Sadly, in many cases lack of guidance led to misdirected study and much wasted time. It is *not* cheating to ask for guidance from your tutor. Other students in your group are just as capable of seeking such help for themselves. Your teachers are resources just as are libraries.

In Chapter 4, I shall discuss problems that arise in the presentation of written assignments, including seen essays. One of the topics covered is the 'academic style' preferred when writing an essay or project for your college.

> It is *not* cheating to ask for guidance from your tutor about a set essay.

Notes

N o t e s

4 Problems of presentation in written assessments

Key topics

- ■ Writing in an appropriate literary style
- ■ Common problems of presentation, such as:
  - — handwriting
  - — grammar
  - — punctuation

  that may impair the marker's impression of your work

Introduction

Poor grammar and bad spelling will not by themselves fail an essay. But careful spelling, neat handwriting and good grammar will help create a positive impression. They also play an important part in effective, accurate communication, which is an important skill for a health professional.

Good presentation will not hide an essay's lack of substance but shoddy presentation may help to hide your essay's good points. You should aim to achieve both a sound structure and content, and a pleasing and clear presentation.

Handwriting

While some may be able to type essays or use a word processor, other students may not have access to these tools. Also, exam essays will almost certainly be handwritten, so the topic of handwriting has to be addressed.

Let me repeat – you don't fail an assessment because of untidy handwriting. Nevertheless, you create a problem if your marker cannot read something you've written.

Your college may include in its marking scheme a small percentage of marks for aspects of written work such as handwriting (see Ch. 3). Its assessment regulations may also cover the occasion when a student's written work cannot be read by the marker. Such regulations may include having the handwritten assessment professionally typed (at the student's expense) before being marked. Presumably, if neither the marker nor the typist can read the assessment, it will gain no marks.

If your handwriting is poor, then the beginning of your course is the time to attempt to do something about it. Bearing in mind that this book is not a handwriting manual, I make the following suggestions:

1. Consider changing the pen you use. Some cheap fountain pens and ballpoints leave blobs of ink on the paper which can then be smeared by your hand or cuff. Use a tissue to wipe the tip of a ballpoint before your begin to write. Typically, pens which cost a lot don't tend to smudge.

   Your pen may have a nib or a ballpoint which is too broad or fine for your particular handwriting. It might be worth experimenting with points or nibs of differing widths in order to find one that suits you.

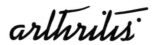

Figure 4.1A
Misplaced dots and cross-strokes.

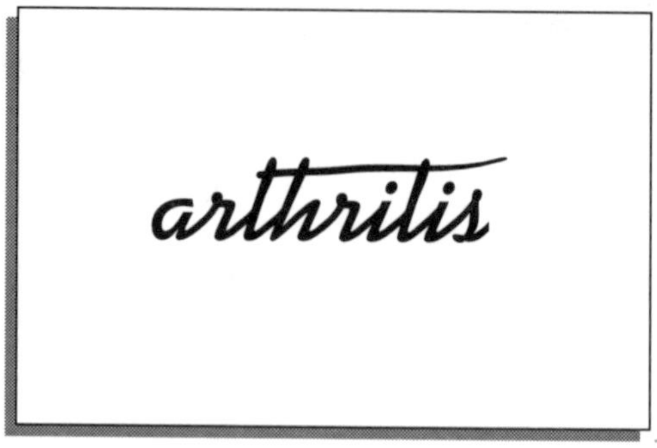

Figure 4.1B
The long cross-stroke that unnecessarily joins all the 't's.

2. Almost inevitably when writing an essay by hand, mistakes occur. (This is where word processors come into their own.) You can use a white correction fluid to cover your mistake, but be sure not to put it on too thickly and to let it dry thoroughly before writing over it. Crossing out your mistake is simpler and quicker (especially important in an exam) so just put *one* stroke of your pen through the mistake, and follow it by the correct version. Your marker will ignore what you have crossed out, even though it may still be legible.

3. Try and analyse your writing to spot any problem areas. Looking at a sample of my own, I found two obvious faults in the way I dot an 'i' and cross a 't' (Fig. 4.1A). The dot above each 'i' is misplaced, usually to the right, and sometimes the 't' is crossed equally inaccurately.

   It would take just a couple of seconds simply to slow down as these danger points approached during writing – to pause, consider, and then cross the 't' or dot the 'i' with greater care. This won't improve my handwriting in total, but it will be a small contribution to making it clearer.

   A related problem occurs where a word contains two or more 't's, and the temptation is to draw a long line which crosses both or all the 't's (Fig. 4.1B). The trouble with this practice is that other letters tend to get in the way. Again pause, think, and add the cross stroke to each individual 't'.

If your own handwriting presents such obvious, yet easily remedied faults, use every opportunity to practise the improved version. By this I mean not just essays written for assessments, but practice essays and the notes you make when reading books and articles. The hope is that it will become second nature to use the improved features when writing by hand, thus taking one small step towards a neater presentation.

Paragraphs

Look at any article in print or a page in a book and you will see, most of the time, that the text has been organized into paragraphs. You'll see that either there is a whole blank line separating paragraphs from each other, or the beginning of a fresh paragraph has been indented (moved slightly from the left hand margin).

The purpose of paragraphs is, briefly, to separate different ideas, and in this way they help to present clearly the structure of the prose. I'll be discussing paragraphs in more detail in Chapter 5. At this stage it is worth saying that paragraphs help to break up a page into smaller-sized chunks, ones that the reader feels are more easily handled. The reverse is also true – when I receive an essay which contains no paragraphs, each page is a mass of words, like a garden so stuffed full of plants you

ADVANTAGES OF USING A WORD PROCESSOR

There is little comparison between using a typewriter and a word processor. The latter allows you to edit as you write, to delete words or whole sentences, to swap the order in which the paragraphs appear, and to correct spelling errors. If you take out a sentence or a word, the text on either side will close up. It you insert a sentence, the text on either side will make way for it. All the changes you wish to make can be viewed on screen before you print out your document, hence saving paper.

Depending on the word processor program and its printer, different 'fonts' can be incorporated in your text – print of varying size, text which is written in italics, underlined, or in bold. However, there is a temptation if you are new to word processing to try out every facility available on your machine, and this can lead to a page which appears fussy and unclear. Stick to one particular device for emphasizing a word – italics, bold, or underlining. Be consistent, too, in the way you set out headings and subheadings.

As you write your document, save it on your disk at frequent intervals. In the event of a power cut, everything you've written that hasn't been saved will vanish – you will have no choice but to write it out again. The word processor's golden rule is: save it! Also keep a back up disk, in case your first disk is damaged.

If possible, get used to your processor before your course begins, or at least before you are set written assessments. Writing an essay for a fast approaching deadline is not the best time to learn how to use your machine. When writing assessments you need to be able to concentrate on your message, not on the machinery for producing it.

Some writers claim that using a word processor makes for a careless writer. Devotees of the word processor will doubtless disagree. Students using typewriters, knowing how much hard work is entailed in rewriting their script, will probably ponder more deeply each sentence they type, than the user of a word processor who knows he can easily change whatever appears on the screen. Conversely, with a word processor it is easier to get something, anything, down in writing, thus escaping from the awful sight of a blank sheet of paper (or a blank screen).

---

can't see any soil in between. An essay which uses paragraphs appears less intimidating, and so goes some way to creating that positive initial impression you want.

Paragraphs give the impression (rightly or wrongly) that the writer has made an attempt to organize his or her thoughts, that the essay has been *planned*.

Grammar and style

Just as this book isn't a handwriting manual, neither is it a textbook of English grammar. Students do not lose marks for bad grammar in their written assessments, any more than they do for poor spelling or untidy handwriting. Sometimes, however, grammatical mistakes can make a difference to the sense of what the student is trying to say. A double negative, for example, gives the opposite meaning to that intended:

■ *'Mr Smith didn't have no pain.'*

Here the patient, through not having 'no pain', must have had *some* pain.

Colleges of health studies should not be called on to teach English grammar to students who have survived 12 or more years of education without noticeably benefitting from them. However, tutors can be faced with written work which is, in its grammar, punctuation and spelling, of a poor quality. How can the student avoid this?

One suggestion is that reading quality newspapers will help students to gain not just facts about, for example, social trends, but also an appreciation of good clear English. It is worth reading an article about poverty, not just to garner the facts but to see how the writer has presented them. Are there long, complex sentences, for example? Or is the article written in such a simple, direct way that it is all the more powerful for that?

Wide reading, for your course and for recreation, will, I believe, bring about an appreciation of what is and what is not good English. You will learn to dismiss the pomposity of using longer words than are necessary, where meaning takes a rear seat to style.

Sometimes difficult words are necessary because, in your chosen health care setting, they have specific meanings and are thus informative. Nurses refer to a patient as 'pyrexial' or as having 'haematuria', neither being words which would commonly be used in everyday conversation. To use long, unusual words for nothing except effect is not, however, the mark of a good communicator.

ACTIVITY

Try this exercise. Read the following short passage – are you impressed by it? Are you amazed at the writer's grasp of English? You shouldn't be – it was invented by me to demonstrate what I've referred to earlier as pomposity. In fact, the passage could be rewritten more simply, and with fewer words. Try and do this yourself.

■ *Surreptitiously did I cast a glance, under cover of the financial pages of my established choice of daily news medium, towards the wall-mounted timepiece, affixed there doubtless in an earlier age by some worthy artisan about his honest business.*

It was but a few minutes before the fifth hour, that time at which I habitually vacated my office and conveyed myself by automobile to my richly furnished apartment on the pastoral fringes of suburbia. I acquainted my colleagues, whose lot it was to accompany me in the daily travail and tedium of gainful employment, with my intention to leave both my chair and their company, albeit at an earlier time than was customary or, indeed, than they might have anticipated.

What did you make of this? The passage could be cut by varying amounts depending on which details you considered were important. Is it necessary, for instance, to include how richly the writer's apartment is furnished, or where it is situated? Does it matter who put the 'timepiece' (or clock) on the wall?

The basic message of these 120 or so words is, 'I decided to go home early'. Even with a few more details included, you could still reduce this to, 'I looked at the clock, and told the people in my office I was going home early.'

A guiding rule to help you avoid such a long-winded style is: set out to *inform*, not to impress your reader(s). When marking students' essays, I sometimes have the impression that the writer is trying desperately hard to impress me by scattering long words over the page, and by constructing lengthy sentences with chains of subordinate clauses and phrases. Often this simply doesn't work, and the lengthier the sentence the less 'punch' it contains. Listen to a politician's answer when he is being interviewed – the longer and more complex the sentence, the likelier it is he is trying to avoid answering the question.

You may have heard of something called the 'academic style'. Perhaps you've already had to write essays or projects using it in an earlier course. It can sound a bit frightening and difficult to achieve at first. There are two aspects of this style that I'll mention here.

A simple prose style is often the most effective.

First is the avoidance of the first person singular – 'I' and 'me'. The academic style's preference is for 'the writer' or 'the present writer'. This gives the prose an air of detachment rather than involvement. Look at the following:

■ Sentence 1. *I discovered from my questionnaire that patients nursed on the intensive care unit were more likely to develop pressure sores than those nursed on my own surgical ward.*

Here the first person singular is used, and not only 'I' but also the possessive 'my' which especially suggests that the writer is somewhat involved in her subject. It is preferable to write in a detached way in your assignments.

■ Sentence 2. *The writer's questionnaire demonstrated that patients nursed on the intensive care unit were more likely to develop pressure sores than those nursed on a surgical ward.*

Both 'I' and 'my' are avoided here. The feeling of the sentence is, I think, undeniably more detached than that of Sentence 1. Sentence 3 is an example of the passive mode, rather than the active:

■ Sentence 3. *It was found that patients nursed on the intensive care unit were more likely to develop pressure sores than those nursed on a surgical ward.*

Here, there is no mention of the person who did the 'finding', neither 'I' nor 'the writer'.

If you're still a little unclear about the active and passive modes here are two more sentences for comparison:

■ Active: *Sister, I'm afraid I've reversed into your new BMW.*
■ Passive: *Sister, I'm afraid your new BMW has been reversed into.*

In the passive sentence, the 'reverser' seems to be distancing himself, understandably, from the scene of the crime, by not mentioning the identity of the reverser.

Interestingly, the accepted use of the third person singular (e.g. 'the writer') in the so-called academic style has been challenged by Burnard, one of Britain's most respected and influential nurse academics and writers. He asks pointedly, 'Who, if not "I", is writing these words?' (Burnard 1994, p. 41). He asserts that many prospective nurse authors strive to use the, to them, unaccustomed third person because they believe it to be an absolute requirement of the academic style. Without this feature, their submission will not be accepted by the editor. So it is with students in colleges of health, required to use the third person by tutors and curriculum planners who insist it is a vital part of the 'correct' academic style. That someone of Burnard's stature thinks otherwise is, to say the least, cause for reflection and reconsideration.

One point Burnard's article fails to make, though, is that the use of the third person singular in an essay or project does help towards creating a detached style – which I consider to be a sound aim for such written work. It is in the more informal, personal viewpoint articles that I frequently have published in *Nursing Standard*, that the first person – I, me, my – is not only permissible but almost indispensable.

A second aspect of the academic style is its apparent reluctance to state things straight out. It appears cautious, overly cautious you might think, and it never seems to state anything as a clear undisputed fact. You would not find the following sentence in a piece of academic writing:

■ *'Nursing standards on the intensive care unit were so poor that, within just two days of their admission, 50% of its patients developed pressure sores.'*

This may be the writer's belief but she would be unwise to write it in such a manner.

Here is my suggestion for how an 'academic writer' might express the same findings:

■ *'Results showed that, of the patients admitted to the intensive care unit, 50% developed pressure sores by the end of the second day. The study suggested that, of a number of possible causative factors, inadequate nursing interventions could be regarded as contributing to these results.'*

In this new version of the earlier statement, there is a clear difference between what is stated as a fact and what is stated as a suggestion. It is a *fact* that 50% of the patients in the unit developed pressure sores. (Perhaps the imaginary study from which this statement might have come provided a definition for precisely what constituted a pressure sore.) It is not, however, a fact that inadequate nursing care caused them, however likely this might seem. Instead, the study *suggests* that inadequate nursing might have *contributed* to the development of sores – among other possible factors. See also how the nursing interventions are described as 'inadequate' rather than 'poor' or 'dreadful'.

Note that the academic writer does not use expressions of emotional involvement. She would not write, for example, 'sadly, 50% patients developed . . .', or 'these appalling results . . .' The researcher may well have a gut feeling that these pressure sores were caused by downright bad nursing, but gut feelings are not admissible in a piece of academic writing.

ACTIVITY

You might like to discuss with your fellow students how difficult or not it could be to write using an academic style. How problematic might it be not to become involved with, or excited by, something you've studied, or at least to avoid the excitement or horror showing through in your writing? Is it acceptable, do you think, to continue using an academic style when writing essays about, say, infant mortality, hypothermia in the elderly, or the sexual abuse of children?

Using the academic style allows you to express *exactly* what has been discovered or what has happened in a research study – hence their expression as 'suggestions' rather than wide generalizations. Asserting something in forthright language does not turn it into an indisputable fact.

Turn to a professional journal such as *Nursing Standard* and compare the articles published there under both the 'Viewpoint' and 'Clinical' labels. Each has its own editor and its own style. Look, too, at one of the 'Occasional Papers' published by *Nursing Times* for a very sound example of an academic style. Can you spot those features of style that suggest detachment?

Punctuation

Again, this book does not set out to be a textbook of punctuation. Just as with previous topics, such as handwriting, I can only give hints about some of the aspects of punctuation that I've found particularly trouble students when they present written work. These are:

● exclamation mark
● apostrophe
● inverted commas (speech marks).

Perhaps it is appropriate to begin with the **exclamation mark** since it does not sit comfortably with the academic style of writing we've just discussed. Exclamation marks may suit certain forms of fiction:

■ *'You swine!' she cried, and pulled from her handbag a submachine gun. 'Take that!'*

Sentences such as these do not fit the academic style at all, even if you found yourself writing a sentence such as:

■ *These results from the questionnaire were completely unexpected.*

An exclamation mark here would make the sentence sound somewhat jovial and light-hearted (and hence intellectually lightweight). The best rule is: if in doubt, don't use an exclamation mark! And above all, *never* use two or three of them!!!

This does not mean that touches of humour have to be rigorously excluded from your written work. Far from it. Look at the following brief passage:

■ *The results from the questionnaire were consistent – but also unexpected. All our respondents' views, from whichever ward situation, matched each others'. The writer had no option but to return to the drawing board.*

I feel that the 'drawing board' term is lightly humorous – there being no actual drawing board – without sounding out of place. Indeed, it shows the writer as being very human and aware of his humanity. A chuckle is all that is called for here, not a belly laugh. Exclamation marks in the passage above would, I believe, have spoiled its effect.

Apostrophes are tricky objects, and in my experience as a marker I've noticed that most students handle the problem by ignoring it altogether and hoping it won't matter. Apostrophes serve two purposes, one of which has already been demonstrated in this paragraph – showing where a letter has been omitted from a word.

Shortening "I have" to "I've", and "will not" to "won't" is acceptable in everyday conversation and in informal texts like this one. But you would tend not to use these forms in an academic essay or study.

A second purpose served by the apostrophe is to denote the possessive. Here, however, the apostrophe can be placed either before or after the letter "s". Compare these sentence groups:

1. a. Here are the books belonging to the student.
   b. Here are the student's books.
2. a. Here are the books belonging to the students.
   b. Here are the students' books.

Where there is only one student (that is, the noun is *singular*) the apostrophe comes before (precedes) the "s":

   "the student's books".

Where there are two or more students (that is, the noun is *plural*) the apostrophe follows the "s":

   "the students' books".

The number of books ('book' being the object of each of the above clauses and phrases) is irrelevant here. So:

   "the student's book" (one student, one book)
   "the students' book" (more than one student, but still only one book).

There is a complication where a word or name ends with an "s". How do you make such a word possessive? Fowler – the bible of English writers – states that formerly (and still in poetry) the name ending with an "s" added the apostrophe only, rather than the apostrophe plus an "s":

"St James . . . St James' Church"

But nowadays, the apostrophe would be followed by a further "s", thus increasing the number of syllables:

"Mr Jones . . ." ("Jones" has only one syllable)
"Mr Jones's hat" ("Jones's" now has two syllables).

Unfortunately, there is another complication. We saw earlier how an apostrophe can denote a missing letter, as in I'm, you're, I'd. This also applies to "it is", which can be reduced, in an informal text, to "it's". But you should note that "it's" does *not* denote a possessive. The possessive form is "its", as in:

"the dog's lead . . . its lead".

So here an apostrophe "s" doesn't signify the possessive.

It is unlikely that missing out apostrophes will make a disastrous difference to the meaning you intend in your essay. It is my view, however, that if students are set a written assessment, it should be as accurate as possible – and this applies as much to the language it's written in as to its clinical detail.

It is also my view that teachers, when marking written assessments, should correct every grammatical error or misspelling. Similarly, teachers' own written comments should be free from such mistakes.

Research has shown that poor standards of written English exist in nursing schools and universities of other English-speaking countries besides the United Kingdom, 'with ramifications for public safety and professional growth' (Hardy et al 1993).

Here is something to think about: some English students, studying a foreign language, were refused the opportunity to participate in a letter exchange scheme with foreign students. This was not because their knowledge of the foreign language was poor, but because their own written English was so bad that the overseas students would not learn from it.

Inverted commas, as you'll have seen throughout this book, are used to denote both someone's speech, and quotations from another writer. You should ascertain whether your college asks for single inverted commas ('...') or double ("...").

WRITING FOR PUBLICATION

In the event of your writing for publication, you should discover which is the preferred 'house style' of your chosen journal or publisher. Getting it right is just one step towards making a favourable impression with your submitted typescript.

It is usual to use single inverted commas, though a little earlier you may have noticed that I changed to double so as not to get you mixed up between inverted commas and apostrophes (as in "Jones's"). A quotation might be inserted into your text thus:

■ *As Smith rightly points out, 'Most preoperative advice provided by nurses is of limited value.'*

Double quotation marks ("...") are usually reserved for quotations inside quotations. This tends to happen less frequently in an academic essay than in fiction, where one of the characters starts to quote another. The writer then has to remember to conclude *both* sets of quotation marks:

■ *She said, 'I will never forget the way he told me, "I love you dearly"'.*

In this example both sets of speech marks end at the same point.

In an essay, be wary of scattering inverted commas around straightforward words just because you want them to be stressed a little. Sometimes I've found passages such as this in students' essays:

■ *When the nurse empties the patient's "bottle" she should make sure to enter the "amount" on his "fluid chart". This is Very Important.*

None of these inverted commas is necessary, and nor are the capital letters for those last two words. To stress one particular word, simply underline it.

WRITING FOR PUBLICATION

Should you write for publication using a typewriter or printer that cannot create italic script, you can underline those words or phrases you want italicized in print. This is a sign to the editor and printer of your wishes. There are many more specialized proof correcting marks used in publishing, and your editor will notify you of those preferred by your journal or publishing house.

Spelling, and meaning what you write

The following collection of words – you would hardly call it a sentence – was taken from an essay I marked a few years ago. How many marks do you think it is worth?

■ *a. fer any patent entering the acccdent and emergency. departement thrers three main priopities are AIRWAY, Breathing a.nd curculation*

This shows how problematic a marker's task can be. It is just possible to squeeze one or two marks out of this assemblage, but there is little to show logical thought and clinical awareness.

Intelligent reading is a well-tried way of improving both your spelling and vocabulary. Read carefully, with a notepad and pencil by you. Don't assume that you can deduce the meaning of a word from its context. Jot down any words you're

USING A SPELLCHECKER

Most word processing programs include a built-in dictionary against which the text you write can be compared for misspellings. Please note, though, that *a spellchecker does not replace an English dictionary.*

Your spellchecker will not tell you the meanings of a word. Nor will it pick out a word that, correctly spelled, is the wrong word for the context in which it occurs.

For example, if you write: 'The patients were asked for ther ages,' the spellchecker will pick out THER for correction. But if you write, 'The patients were asked for there ages,' the spellchecker will not highlight THERE because, even though it is the wrong word, it is nevertheless a correctly spelled English word that occurs in the program's built-in dictionary.

Word processor dictionaries tend not to include technical or specialist words. If you write a word such as 'tachycardia' the spellchecker will probably pick it out as misspelled. It isn't, of course, but it is simply too specialist for your spellchecker's dictionary. Some programs enable you to build up your own specialist dictionary, so that you can enter, say, nursing terminology as you use it in your work. As this specialist dictionary increases in size, fewer correctly spelled words will be picked out as misspelled. But you will *still* need an English dictionary!

not sure about, and check their meaning in a dictionary, such as the Pocket Oxford or Collins. Some dictionaries specialize in contemporary English or technical and scientific terms. You'll also come across dictionaries of psychology and sociology, and dictionaries for nurses.

Don't *misuse* words. Look at the following short sentences:

- *He was literally boiling over with rage.*
- *The nursing staff has been decimated by 'flu.*

You may think there's nothing wrong with these, especially the first. We often use the word 'literally' to mean 'very'. If you're not certain what it means, look it up. Then ponder whether it is humanly possible for someone literally to boil over, or to be literally green with envy.

'Decimate' has an exact meaning, and it is highly unlikely that 'flu will have destroyed exactly one tenth of the nursing staff. (Some large dictionaries, such as Collins, contain interesting notes on the use and misuse of words like 'literally'.)

Use words with care – that is the message here. It is especially important in health care, where words are often used to communicate exact meanings. As an example, a drug can be referred to as an 'agonist', and another as an 'antagonist'. The words sound very similar, but they have opposite meanings.

- *The patient should be placed on the Glasgow Coma Scale to prevent injury.*

Here is another somewhat ludicrous example taken from a student's essay. There are two errors here. First of all, observing a patient using the Glasgow Coma Scale as a tool will not prevent injury. The head injury has already occurred. The Glasgow Scale is used to detect any changes in neurological signs *following* injury.

The second error is one that commonly occurs in essays:

- *The patient is placed on a fluid balance chart.*

Please note that this is not one of those 'howlers' (were they ever funny?) such as the patient being 'under the doctor'. It is more serious than that. It demonstrates a misunderstanding of the point of nursing care.

The *point* of care is not to fill in a chart, whether it is 'placed under the patient' or at the foot of the bed. The point is to complete certain observations on your patient which are then recorded on the proper chart. Do you see the difference? A student's essay which simply mentions a particular chart or scale doesn't convince me, as marker, that he or she knows the principle of care. But:

- *The patient's urine output is recorded on his fluid balance chart, together with the amount of fluid he drinks each day. This is to ensure the patient is correctly hydrated.*

Yes, it does take longer to write. But it demonstrates a better awareness of care than does tucking coma scales and fluid charts underneath the patient – and consequently it earns more marks.

Using abbreviations

As a general rule, it is unacceptable to incorporate abbreviations within your essay or project unless you first provide the full version. In some earlier examples, I used the phrase 'intensive care unit' several times. This takes quite a few key strokes on a word processor or, in an exam, several valuable seconds to write out in full. If,

> When reading, always check the meanings of words you don't know.

however, I give the term's abbreviations in brackets after its first appearance, I can then continue using the abbreviations only. For example:

■ *Over 50 patients involved in road traffic accidents (RTAs) were admitted to the intensive care unit (ICU) during 1994, an increase of 22% from 1993. This was not, however, accompanied by a comparable increase in ICU nurses.*

Furthermore, the rise in incidence of serious RTA casualties was matched by a similar rise (20%) in severe self-poisoning cases, which likewise required admission to ICU.

A number of points should be noted from this brief passage. First, although the abbreviation 'ICU' rightly appears in capital letters, lower case letters are used for the phrase in full ('intensive care unit'). Second, having established 'ICU' as your preferred term, don't then swap between it and 'ITU' (meaning 'intensive therapy unit', an alternative term used by some hospitals). Third, in the first abbreviation used in the example, you'll have noticed that, although 'RTA' appears in capital letters, the final 's' is lower case. Can you work out why? (It's because that final 's' isn't part of the abbreviated term but simply denotes the plural. You will find the same when you come across the abbreviation for non-steroidal antiinflammatory drugs – NSAIDs.)

One problem with using abbreviations in an essay is that your reader might not be familiar with their meaning, or might know of a different meaning to that you intend. That is why it is so important to provide the full term first, so that your reader (and marker) knows exactly what you mean. Some forms of abbreviation simply look sloppy as in this example from a student's rushed exam answer:

■ *The patient was seen by the dr and prescribed pain killers.*

There is probably little doubt what is meant here, but that 'dr' doesn't enhance the appearance of the essay, and so is best avoided. As a sound general rule, don't use abbreviations in academic written work unless you show their meaning clearly.

Finally – the battle of the sexes

There is one more problem I want to discuss about the presentation of your written assessments: how to use male and female pronouns.

The majority of nurses are female, as are the majority of occupational therapists and physiotherapists. But there are male nurses and male therapists, as well as female surgeons and physicians. Patients are likewise both female and male.

In the past, textbooks, particularly of nursing, would mostly use 'she' for the nurse and 'he' for the patient (except where the latter was necessarily female). Some textbooks began with a brief note explaining that this practice was adopted for clarity – others did not.

As a male student nurse I was often offended by words which embraced us all, metaphorically speaking, as being one gender. Then I discovered that female medical students felt the same way about continually being referred to as 'he' in medical texts.

Words matter. You do not have to go to the more bizarre extremes of political correctness to use a system which accepts that both males and females may be nurses, therapists, doctors and patients.

Personally, I dislike the clumsiness of using 's/he', and even 'he or she' (or 'she or he') is somewhat long-winded. Until a gender-neutral pronoun is invented and comes into common usage you will have to make do with what is now available.

(Incidentally, my suggestion for gender-neutral pronouns is 'ge' for he/she and 'gir' for him/her, with the letter 'g' pronounced gutterally, as in Dutch. I wonder if it will catch on?)

You could begin your assignment with a disclaimer (doctors and patients are 'he', nurses and therapists are 'she') but I think this is nowadays unacceptable.

The method I've chosen in this book is simply to use different personal pronouns at different points. So on one page a nurse may be male, while two pages later the nurse is female. Likewise the therapists 'swap' genders. There is no system – I don't count up the male and female pronouns to see if they match. I do feel, however, that this way you avoid any literary eyesores like s/he. Discussion with your teachers and among your colleagues may help you make your mind up about what is best. If your college has a required method, it should be drawn to your attention by your teacher.

In Chapter 5 I shall discuss the importance of your essays having a structure. I'll also be adding to what I've already said in this chapter about the use of paragraphs.

REFERENCES

Burnard P 1994 Keep it simple. Nursing Standard 8 (34): 41
Hardy L, Seagore M , Edge D 1993 Illiteracy: implications for nursing education. Nurse Education Today 13, 24–29

USEFUL READING

Fowler H W 1983 A dictionary of modern English usage. Oxford University Press, Oxford
Weiner E S C, Hawkins J M 1984 The Oxford guide to the English language. Oxford University Press, Oxford
Churchill Livingstone 1989 Nurses' dictionary, 16th edn. Churchill Livingstone, Edinburgh

Plus
A recent edition of a good English dictionary:
e.g. The Pocket Oxford Dictionary, The Shorter Collins Dictionary

5 Structuring an essay

■ The significance of an essay's structure to its logic and argument
■ How structure may be achieved and demonstrated to the reader
■ Important checks to make to your essay before its final submission

Introduction – the significance of structure

If you are a painter, it is likely that you will understand the importance of structure in your own pictures. You will ensure that one side of your canvas is not crowded with figures, trees and buildings, while the other is left empty.

Similarly with music. The great majority of pre-20th century concerti, symphonies and sonatas have movements which are built on a particular structure. A listener without musical training may not be aware of this, but he will almost certainly feel a sense of rightness when, towards the end of a movement, its main theme returns.

So it is with writing. If you are fond of crime novels, you will be well used to the structure adopted by most novelists – the setting, the sleuth, the deed, the suspects' interviews, the final revelation. You would feel cheated if the murderer's identity is revealed to be someone who has played no part in the rest of the book.

All these examples of structure within various art forms are similar in that the structure plays a major part in establishing the viewers', listeners', or readers' satisfaction with the piece, whether consciously or not. Form is as vital to an essay as to a picture.

Structure is the framework on which you hang your argument, turning your essay from a succession of unconnected sentences into an ordered and logical discussion. Like a house, your essay has a front door (the introduction) and a back door (the conclusion) and its foundations are the data derived from your search of the literature and, perhaps, your clinical experience.

Features of an essay's structure

An essay's structure will vary according to its subject and treatment, but there are some common features.

The title

First of all there will be an informative title. I shall discuss titles again in a later chapter, but here it is simply necessary to say that your title should illuminate your essay's subject. You may have been asked to formulate a title (perhaps on a given subject) or your college may have given you and your colleagues a set title. If the latter, it will have been rigorously discussed by your college's assessment committee or examinations board in order to iron out any problems or shades of meaning which could confuse students.

Lengthy, informative titles are preferable for an academic essay, rather than punchy, attention-grabbing titles favoured by fiction writers. Thus a title such as, 'Differences in the perception of patients' pain by house officers and registered nurses' is preferable to 'What's up doc?'

Where you are given a choice of essay title, you should take care to show which choice you have made. It is unwise to require your marker to guess, from your answer, which topic you have chosen.

The abstract

It is not always necessary for abstracts to be written for essays, and your teacher will tell you if this is the case for yours. Where a longer piece of work, such as a project or special study, is being written, or if you are submitting an academic piece to a professional journal, an abstract is usually required.

Journal editors, and your college's assessment regulations, will usually specify how long an abstract should be – 200 words is about the usual size. Your abstract should summarize the essay's content, and because your word count is so limited you should restrict yourself to principal points only.

The introduction

If your essay word limit is, say, 3000 words, you should set yourself a sensible word limit for its introduction, such as 400 to 500 words. Doing this, you avoid ending up with an unbalanced piece of work – heavy on introducing the topic, but light on actually discussing it.

You may use part of the introduction for explaining your choice of essay topic (if you were offered a choice) and for setting out useful definitions. In writing about your choice of subject, it is perhaps acceptable to resort to 'I' and 'my' despite this being an academic essay. Look at the following brief example:

■ *One of my clinical placements was based in a health centre on a run down council estate in Anytown. Here, while working with a team of district nurses, I saw examples of how ill health may have been attributable to poor diet and health education. Visiting some of the homes in the estate's tower blocks, I witnessed further examples of damp, inadequately heated flats, and families that were terrified of over-spending on food and heat beyond their state benefits.*

In every case it was the mother who took charge of the family's meagre finances and, consequently, bore the brunt of stress, feelings of guilt, and manifestations of failing health. I almost felt as if I had no choice except this particular essay title – that it, in fact, chose me.

What do you think of this? It is a purely imaginary introduction and you may feel it goes 'over the top'. You may feel it places its mythical writer far too close to her subject. Yet somehow it brings the chosen subject to life for me. It also suggests that the student will set out to establish links between her clinical placements and what she has read in her college library. It *is* a very personal introduction, and doubtless the 'meat' of the essay would have to be written in a more detached manner, but it by no means reads like a tabloid. Rather, it shows a concerned awareness, and an interest in the chosen topic, and as such I would applaud it.

If this introduction were for an essay on, say, the link between poverty and ill health, part of the opening paragraphs could be devoted to the problems of defining poverty. This then forges a clear link with the main body of your essay in which you discuss, say, three definitions of poverty, examining their good and bad points.

Alternatively, your introduction might set the scene by describing the council estate mentioned above. This is where the alleged poverty exists, you say; this is where the team of district nurses works. Later in your essay you could draw links between the theories of poverty, as derived from the literature, and your field experience.

However you choose to introduce your essay, you should attempt to show a link between it and what follows. What spoils the 'feel' of an essay is where there is a distinct jolt, a sudden swerve of direction, between the end of the introduction and the opening of the essay's discussion. The introduction must *belong* to the main text that follows it.

The main argument

In marking essays from student nurses, I have noticed two basic common errors. The first is not to pay too much attention to the essay title; the second is to pour forth a flow of words with no thought to planning or structure. Both of these faults could be summarized by an adapted essay title: 'All I know about . . .'.

It is as if the student has glanced at the question and fixed his attention on one or two obvious words or phrases. Look at this example of an adult nursing essay topic:

■ *'Discuss how effective nursing assessment of a patient during her admission to your ward may enhance the patient's care following routine surgery.'*

This question asks you to forge links between patient assessment and postoperative care. There is a tendency, however, for some students to fasten onto a couple of familiar phrases – postoperative care, patient admission – and for the essay consequently to be turned into, 'All I know about admitting patients and caring for them after their operation.'

A near perfect description of postoperative care will gain few marks if there is no connection with what happened during the patient's admission. However, a well-planned essay might show that, by taking the patient's temperature during her admission, the nurse is helping to rule out the possibility of an infection which could adversely affect the planned operation. If the student links this particular observation with, say, taking the patient's midstream specimen of urine (in order to rule out a urinary tract infection) extra marks would be gained by putting the assessment procedure into its proper context.

Your essay's structure should be derived from your careful reading of the essay title as it is set, and not as you imagine it to be after a cursory glance.

> Answer the essay title *exactly* as it is written, and not as you adapt it.

ACTIVITY

Can you think of a way of setting out your essay for the above topic? Take a few minutes to jot down some thoughts about the structure of this essay. Don't get too worried about its factual content, because probably there is much that you've not yet covered in your course. Concentrate on its *form*.

The main problem with this essay will probably be how you join the two principal themes – assessment on admission and postoperative care.

What have you come up with? Perhaps you've discussed this exercise with a few of your colleagues – have you found any particularly interesting or innovative ideas?

An obvious way of structuring this essay – but one fraught with danger – is first to describe how a patient is assessed on admission to the ward, and then to describe her care following her operation. The structure of the essay is therefore two large 'blocks' of text. I've tried to show this in Figure 5.1A. In order to link the two blocks, during the second part of the essay you could incorporate what might be called 'flashbacks', which draw links with the first block.

As an example, you could write, 'The patient's pulse and blood pressure are taken hourly on her return to the ward from theatre.' And then comes the 'flashback' or link, 'The patient's pulse and blood pressure recorded during her admission to the

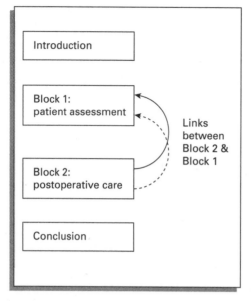

Figure 5.1A
A simple essay structure – two main blocks of text with links between Block 2 and Block 1.

Figure 5.1B
An essay structure showing clear links between patient assessment and postoperative care.

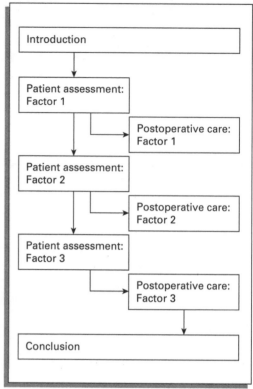

ward act as a baseline so that, after the operation, the nurse can assess any significant changes in these observations.'

I'm sure you will have noticed the possible dangers. The first is that the student writes 'Block 1', a description of patient assessment, without any reference to (and so perhaps without any thought for) 'Block 2'. It is only when the student describes postoperative care that links between the two blocks are made. It would be all too possible to carry on writing, providing the marker with 'all I know about postoperative care' while neglecting to show these vital links. The two blocks end up disparate and detached, like two monolithic skyscrapers. A second danger is that the student, through failing to show the necessary links, also fails to *discuss* (which is what the question asked). Instead, his answer consists of simple description – an account of what he actually does. Noting the links between patient assessment and postoperative care would, I think, prompt the student to convert his answer from description to discussion (I shall be examining the meaning of words such as 'discuss' and 'describe' in Chapter 11.)

Another method of structuring your essay is shown in Figure 5.1B. After the introduction, aspects of the nursing assessment of the patient are discussed, one after the other, but with very firm links with the patient's postoperative care *at each step*. Thus, if the student begins the main body of his essay with details of the patient's clinical observations on admission – temperature, pulse, blood pressure and respirations – he can discuss their significance both for this point in her hospital stay

ACTIVITY

You may find it useful to acquire some further essay questions – from differing fields of nursing or therapy – and, in small groups, draw up essay plans showing how you would structure them. If you can, provide alternative structures showing the advantages and disadvantages of each.

and when she is recovering from her operation. The links are there, very obvious, for the marker to see.

Later he may write about assessing the patient's social background (husband, young children, job) and again will show links between this and the communication of important information from the nurse to the husband after the operation is over.

This essay title we've been discussing seeks a thoughtful exposition of nursing care, rather than a James Joycian 'flow of consciousness': everything-I-know-about-patient-care-and-a-bit-more-just-in-case-it-earns-me-some-more-marks.

In this respect, the *structure* of the essay is central to its quality of discussion. Structure is not something tacked on the end; it is a vital component. I have demonstrated its importance using just one essay title.

Conclusion

Just as an effective essay requires an introduction, so it also deserves a well thought out conclusion. It is probably true to say that there is no one right answer to every essay you are set, especially for essays grounded in sociology or social policy. These are best planned as an exposition of differing, and perhaps conflicting, viewpoints. You might, for example, discuss a socialist approach to state welfare benefits contrasted with a Thatcherite approach. You don't have to show that either is the only correct approach (neither is, probably).

Your conclusion will, however, draw together the main points of your argument which you've set down in the main body of your essay. It acts as a reminder of what has gone before, rather like the judge's summing up at the end of a trial for the benefit of the jury. Your conclusion is to help underline the central arguments of your essay to its marker. Thus:

■ *'In this essay I have looked at the changes in welfare benefits from 1979 to 1988, and contrasted the attitude of Mrs Thatcher's government to the concept of the welfare state with that of the preceding socialist regimes.'*

Your conclusion is not the place for additional facts or new arguments. Nor should you repeat any quotations from the literature you incorporated into your main text.

 ACTIVITY

What sort of conclusion would the essay on patient assessment and postoperative care require? Try and draw up a useful summary of what ought to be included – not clinical fine detail but a review of major points made. Your conclusion might begin:

■ *'In this essay it has been shown that accurate individual patient assessment, carried out when the patient is admitted to the ward, forms an effective basis for the safe and empathic care of the patient following surgery.'*

In other words, if in your essay's main text you managed to demonstrate links between patient assessment and postoperative care, your conclusion will draw the reader's attention to those links rather than to individual facets of either assessment or care.

References and bibliography

Your college assessment regulations will tell you whether references are required for the essays you submit. It is likely, however, that they will be. You should note whether a bibiography is also needed.

A concluding list of references includes all those articles and books that your essay actually referred to. Thus, if your essay contained the text: 'Research by Thomas

(1988) showed a clear connection between . . .', then Thomas 1988 should appear in your final Reference section.

It might be, however, that certain texts were found to be very useful as background material to your essay. You read through Brown 1991 and Jones 1992 in order to get your thoughts in order for your essay. They helped you think of a way of structuring your essay and pointed you in the direction of other texts. If your essay didn't actually refer to either Brown 1991 or Jones 1992 – you didn't quote them, nor did you clearly state any of their findings – then these authors would appear in your Bibliography rather than your References section.

Remember that different methods of writing references will be discussed in Chapter 7. It is perhaps worth noting here that an important function of a reference is to allow your reader to follow up the literature that you have found useful. References should be both sufficiently detailed and *accurate*. 'Could a reader go to the text I've used?' is the question you should ask yourself when you write a reference to the literature.

Ways of achieving structure

Having seen earlier how important structure is to a good essay, now is the time to discuss how structure may be achieved and, just as important, demonstrated to your marker. I think it will help me to explain the process of essay construction if I give you a specific essay question:

■ *'Discuss the role of the nurse or therapist as health educator in today's society.'*

I'm going to suggest a series of stages through which the student might work in preparing to write this essay. These stages are:

● brainstorming
● writing prompt cards
● shuffling the pack
● deciding.

Brainstorming

The first stage is brainstorming, an excellent technique for any form of written assessment from essays to longer projects. On a sheet of paper jot down ideas that occur to you while reading your set question. Don't think about these ideas just yet, and don't dismiss any of them as wildly inappropriate. Get them down so that you can study them later.

Brainstorming can usefully be carried out within your student group – many of your ideas will be similar, but sometimes you can achieve a quite different slant on the subject by employing more than one brain.

 ACTIVITY

Perhaps you'd like to do your own brainstorming session now for the essay topic I've given. Try and see if you can arrive at about 20 ideas. To set you off here are a few of my own, ideas that I've not thought about at all but that simply occurred to me as I wrote this passage:

● district nurse
● Project 2000
● accident service
● alcohol
● cigarettes.

Writing prompt cards

Having achieved a good list of ideas, read it through considering each item in turn. Some items will be obviously linked (as could be alcohol and cigarettes in my own brief list above). Some might be all too obviously irrelevant. Using either slips of paper or those 15 cm by 10 cm (6 in by 4 in) record cards I mentioned in Chapter 2, write each item on a separate slip in order to form a 'pack' of ideas.

At this point, using the cards as prompts, you will spend a good time reading up on the essay's subject. The literature you read will undoubtedly give you further ideas so don't hesitate to add these to your pack of cards.

Shuffling the pack

Now comes the stage of 'shuffling the pack', just as I showed in Figure 2.5. Try your ideas in different groupings and in different orders – I'll give you an example of what I mean shortly.

Deciding

Finally, you must decide which order is most appropriate for the essay you want to construct. Now is also perhaps the time to think how your ideas can best be introduced so as to clarify your essay's structure.

Let me return to 'shuffling the pack' and explain what it involves.

It occurs to me that there are several ways of organizing all my ideas for the set question. Here are three of those ways:

1. Using different therapist and nursing groups as the means of organizing my essay:
   - district nurses
   - school nurses
   - health visitors
   - nurses on acute wards
   - nurses on paediatric wards
   - community occupational therapists
   - physiotherapist on an orthopaedic ward.

Do any of my 'ideas pack' fit into each of these categories? Perhaps some will find a logical place under several.

2. Using different health care settings as the means of organizing my essay:
   - primary and secondary schools
   - occupational health departments in industry
   - acute hospital wards
   - outpatient clinics
   - accident service.

You will easily note the similarities between this list and the previous one, but there are differences too. Again, how well do the items in my ideas pack fit under these headings?

3. Using different health education problems as the means of organizing my essay:
   - alcohol use
   - drug and solvent abuse
   - cigarette smoking
   - unhealthy diet
   - AIDS and HIV.

Again, see how all the items in your ideas pack will fit under these and similar headings. I'm sure you will easily think of other headings within each of the above three schemes, and perhaps especially in the third. But, given our essay's word count, it is as well to acknowledge that we must restrict its scope.

I'm going to continue with scheme 3 in order to show how our essay might be organized.

First, I'll use part of the introduction to explain why the range of my essay is going to be limited to a discussion of, say, three areas of concern in health education: cigarette smoking, sexual behaviour, and diet. Your marker won't penalize you because you've omitted to mention solvent or drug abuse, especially if you make it clear from the outset what you are concentrating on, and provided the restriction you have made is admissible within the set essay.

The rest of the introduction could be devoted to a brief overview of recent changes in the health service and, in particular, nurse education, changes which have shifted nursing concerns from an almost total concentration on the diseased body to the support and education of the healthy individual. (Remember those significant words in the essay question: '. . . in today's society.')

Now I'm going to discuss the main body of the essay. If I don't use any specific arrangement of the cards in my ideas pack, my essay could easily degenerate into a succession of sentences, a jumble of ideas, each unconnected to one another. Alternatively, it would be all too easy to fasten on one idea and discuss it interminably, thus omitting all reference to other topics.

The arrangement of my ideas cards that I finally pick as the most suitable, will dictate the essay's structure. This structure is demonstrated, to myself and to the marker, by my use of headings, subheadings and paragraphs.

Using headings

Just as this book, and many other health care texts, uses a system of headings and subheadings, so can your essay. I have heard it said that headings spoil the look of an essay, and consequently its flow of ideas, but such a view escapes me. It is better surely to use a tool that actively clarifies one's writing – and both headings and paragraphs can do just that.

Figure 5.2 shows an outline of my essay, with headings, subheadings and paragraphs. You will appreciate that the number of paragraphs under each subheading will vary, though I have indicated just a limited number. It is important to use a consistent method of print or type for headings and subheadings which are of equal importance. This is illustrated in Figure 5.2, where major headings (Introduction, Cigarette smoking, Sexual activity, etc.) are printed in bold type and underlined, while the lesser subheadings (At school, In industry, etc.) are printed in ordinary type and underlined. You should also be consistent in your use of capital letters. Note that only the first word of each heading and subheading begins with a capital letter.

Does all this sound fussy? Perhaps it does, but I maintain that consistency will help to clarify your essay's structure. Consistency in headings improves not only the appearance of your essay, but the sense it makes.

Incidentally, if you look at Figure 5.2 you'll see one other feature that enhances the structure of this essay outline. Can you spot it? It is the inclusion of 'The nurse's role' as a separate subheading under each main heading. It ensures that you do discuss the role of nursing within each of the problem areas chosen. You may disagree with its position within a separate section. You may prefer to include something about the nurse's role within each subheading – in industry or at school, for example. I have simply shown it as it appears in Figure 5.2 to emphasize its place within the essay's overall structure, and its importance within the essay title itself. It mustn't be forgotten amongst all the other information you want to get across. (Other health care professionals would replace 'nurse' with 'physiotherapist' or 'occupational therapist'. The structure of the essay would work as well for them as for nurses.)

> Be consistent in the appearance of headings and subheadings in your essay.

Using paragraphs

Now, what about the paragraphs that appear under each heading? How is the text of my essay divided into paragraphs?

We saw in an earlier chapter how off-putting is the sight of pages of script

Introduction
      Paragraph 1
      Paragraph 2
Cigarette smoking
    At school
      Paragraph 3
    Government campaigns
      Paragraph 4
    The nurse's role
      Paragraph 5
      Paragraph 6
Sexual activity
    Influence of the media
      Paragraph 7
    Government campaigns
      Paragraph 8
    Voluntary organisations
      Paragraph 9
    The nurse's role
      Paragraph 10
      Paragraph 11
Diet
    School meals
      Paragraph 12
    Fashion diets
      Paragraph 13
    Government campaigns
      Paragraph 14
    The nurse's role
      Paragraph 15
      Paragraph 16
Conclusion

Figure 5.2
Essay plan showing headings, subheadings and paragraphs.

containing no indentations or missed lines, and thus no individual paragraphs. The mass of writing seems to overpower the reader in its bulk. Paragraphs, on the other hand, break up your text, just as the headings do. Paragraphs are an extension of the heading system I've already discussed.

Usually, each paragraph contains an idea, a part of the discussion, which though separate from the other ideas that occur (in the other paragraphs) links with them. Thus paragraphs 5 and 6 in Figure 5.2 could be divided so that, while paragraph 5 discussed the role of the school nurse regarding health education and cigarette smoking, paragraph 6 would deal with the role of the occupational health nurse in industry.

You need to be clear in your mind what the purpose is of each of your paragraphs. In this way, you don't start dodging back and forth between subjects as you remember additional points.

I have said that different paragraphs contain different, though related, ideas. It is important for your essay's structure, and for the ease with which it can be read, that there are smooth transitions between successive paragraphs. Such smoothness helps your reader to follow the argument your essay is trying to develop. Arguments – or critical discussions – don't consist simply of stating facts vehemently (although if you listen to debates from the House of Commons you might believe that to be true). Instead, an argument is constructed by assembling groups of facts (as derived from both the literature and your field or clinical experience) and demonstrating the relationships between those facts. You introduce counterarguments – views that seem to oppose the initial thrust of your assembled facts, and which are also backed up by the literature. Subsequently, you show how one group of facts and the relationships between them make one viewpoint so much more likely than another. This whole argument is carried out in that calm detached manner which is described, rightly or wrongly, as the 'academic style'.

So that this argument can be followed clearly, your reader must be able to move from one paragraph – one stage of the argument – to the next with ease. Ideally, your reader shouldn't lose track at any point or need to retrace his steps to earlier paragraphs to get his bearings. This means the transition from one paragraph (one idea) to the next should not be a literary jolt.

Here is one example where the opening sentence of a new paragraph doesn't seem to match the closing sentence of its predecessor:

■ *District nurses working for inner-city group practices have found themselves assessing elderly patients whose symptoms seem to derive more from their poor living conditions than from any primary disease.*

Tower blocks of flats were initially inhabited by families of all sizes displaced by slum clearances in the 1960s.

You could probably work out a link between these two paragraphs (and remember there is only one sentence for you to consider from each) but it would be possible to devise a far smoother transistion from the end of the first paragraph to the beginning of the next. See what you think of this slight adaptation to the above example:

■ *District nurses working for inner city group practices have found themselves assessing elderly patients whose symptoms seem to derive more from their poor living conditions than from any primary disease.*

Typical of such deprived living conditions are the many tower blocks of flats which, initially inhabited by families of all sizes displaced by slum clearances in the 1960s, are now mostly reserved for the elderly and the single unemployed.

Can you see how this smoother transition has been achieved? You'll probably notice the repeated phrase 'living conditions' present in both paragraphs. Such link phrases needn't be repeated verbatim but, in order to serve their linking purpose, must be recognizable. In my example above, the longer phrase 'poor living conditions' has been purposely (though slightly) altered to 'deprived living conditions'. This tiny alteration itself helps, I think, to move the argument of this imaginary essay forward a little. These link words or phrases can be considered from two directions.

One direction (notice how the word 'direction' provides a link with the previous paragraph) is that of a forward looking 'signpost'. It is a word or phrase occurring at or toward the end of a paragraph which you, the writer, know will recur in the opening sentence of the next. It is a signpost because it is pointing the reader towards the next idea, the next related strand of your developing argument. You, the writer, purposely plant this signpost in the last sentence of your current paragraph, knowing it will point the way to the next.

Instead of using a signpost, however, you can arrange for a certain phrase, occurring in the first sentence of a new paragraph, to glance back over its shoulder, as it were, towards a similar phrase at the end of the preceding paragraph. This method is perhaps slightly easier to handle than the first because, once you've written a satisfactory paragraph (which you are then loathe to alter) and you're about to start the next, you can glance back at the last sentence you wrote and try to derive some phrase from it, or based on it, to begin your new paragraph.

Another method of linking paragraphs, especially if there is to be a change of direction in your argument or discussion, is to use particular linking words or phrases that warn the reader of this change: words and phrases like 'however' and 'by contrast'. You can use certain words and phrases even when there is no change of direction: 'similarly', 'as I have shown', 'as was seen earlier'. Sometimes it can be very effective purposely to create an abrupt change of subject or mood between paragraphs, as if you were deliberately breaking the rules of sound writing practice. Rather like beginning sentences with words such as 'And' or 'But' (which is frowned on) this requires experience of writing and careful technique – and so you'll notice that I haven't attempted to give you an example here.

How structure can help critically

Planning the content and order of paragraphs in an essay helps you achieve the fundamental goal of actually *addressing the essay topic as it is set*. Planning the content of the paragraphs, and arranging the order of their appearance, enables you to *discuss* rather than describe, or to *evaluate critically*, as required by the essay's title. You cannot develop an argument if your subject matter is scattered at random across the essay, written down as ideas pop into your head. Instead, there has to be a logical formation of ideas into paragraphs and an equally logical flow of those ideas from one paragraph to the next, from the essay's planned beginning to its planned conclusion.

Let me try and demonstrate this quality of *criticality* (and its lack) in essay writing, using another essay topic, one that I think will appeal to students of occupational therapy, physiotherapy and nursing equally:

■ *Critically evaluate the changing position of people with physical disabilities from 1975 to 1995.*

Now, this is a subject which I know a bit, since it is one that affects me personally; and therefore there is the risk that I rush into this essay without adequate planning, in order to get down on paper any and every jot of information I know. There is another risk: that my naturally biased views will prompt me to give a lot of space to one side of the argument without an adequate amount of space (or indeed any) to the opposing side. This is a particular danger when you write essays on subjects with which you are passionately involved. There is absolutely nothing wrong with being passionate about a subject, or with hastily jotting down ideas on paper – so long as the latter is an initial brainstorming session rather than writing the essay proper.

So let me try and give you a brief glimpse of what I would consider to be a hasty and ill-planned essay on the above topic. You should assume that the following example occurs within the main section of the essay, after the introduction (if there actually was one):

■ *Access to public buildings has certainly improved over the past 20 years, with more ramps installed in shops, banks and post offices. Disability awareness has been taken on board by the government in 1995, issuing pamphlets concerning how disabled people can be discriminated against. Many new disability benefits were introduced during the 1980s. Some disability groups seem to have become more outspoken, holding demonstrations outside the BBC and ITV television centres, and holding up traffic in Oxford Street, London. The government has introduced an antidiscrimination bill for disabled people in January 1995 following their issuing of a discussion paper in late 1994. A new Incapacity for Work benefit is being brought in in April 1995 which will help those whose ill health and disabilities prevent them from working.*

There is much information here, but it has two important faults. First of all, it is disorganized. Disability benefits, for example, are mentioned twice, though separately. Also situated well apart is mention of both a government-backed antidiscrimination Bill in Parliament, and the production of a disability awareness booklet by the government. Perhaps, too, there could be a link – that of access – between the writer's initial assertion that access has improved over the past 20 years, and demonstrations by disability activists in Oxford Street.

The second principal fault of the passage quoted is that it is almost entirely uncritical. (Bear in mind, however, that to be critical does not mean that you must be *negatively* critical. A critical appraisal can be highly positive, if that is appropriate to the facts you present.) The writer mentions the creation of new benefits without noting which existing benefits they replaced, and to what effect. In the case of Incapacity for Work benefit, the writer could have pointed out that this will be subject to income tax, which the replaced Invalidity Benefit was not, and that it is accessed by new stringent medical assessment. The writer could have mentioned that, while physical access to many public buildings is possible in 1995, wheelchair users still have no right of access to polling stations at election time, and so have restricted voting rights. The writer could have drawn links between the production by the current government of leaflets on disability awareness, and the perceived need for activists to demonstrate outside ITV and BBC television centres. Why were they demonstrating? Did it have to do with the broadcasting of charity programmes to which some people object? Finally, while there is mention of antidiscrimination legislation in 1995, nothing is said about the dozen or so attempts at more stringent legislation, promoted by backbenchers, during the preceding 10 or so years.

I hesitate to provide you with a 'model answer', my own improved version of the earlier disorganized passage, because it will doubtless be subject to readers' closest examination in order to prove it somewhat less than 'model'! However, below I give you paragraph headings relating to just one aspect of disability issues, that might have been included in a well-organized essay. This single aspect is the (apparent) need for antidiscrimination legislation. I hope you'll be able to see, just from the brief headings, how these few paragraphs are well organized, and have the potential of affording critical discussion:

- **Paragraph 1:** an overview of disability discrimination in Britain, and why legislation is needed
- **Paragraph 2:** details of the 1995 antidiscrimination Bill in regard to
  — employment of disabled adults
  — access to public transport by disabled passengers
  — suitable housing for families with a disabled member
- **Paragraph 3:** a comparison of the earlier (1994) backbencher's Bill (the 'Berry Bill') in regard to the above three subject areas
- **Paragraph 4:** a comparison with the Americans with Disabilities Act 1990, and its effect on the lives of disabled citizens in the USA
- **Paragraph 5:** the costs of the 1995 Bill in its implication for British industry, compared with the costs estimated to arise from the Berry Bill
- **Paragraph 6:** an estimation of how the 1995 Bill, once passed through Parliament, will influence both public awareness and the daily lives of disabled people.

Such a detailed examination of one topic – out of the many possible topics related to disability issues that could have been chosen – obviously requires an acknowledgement in the essay's introduction that only one or two topics have been chosen for critical analysis. (A related subject might be that of disability awareness among the general public, or within the media.) I would say, however, that limiting the scope of your essay in this manner, while striving to achieve depth and criticality of discussion, is preferable to the earlier example I showed of random, uncritical jottings. I hope I have also shown how planning your essay in advance is a vital step in achieving a good grade for a worthy effort and a worthwhile essay.

Planning your essay means being clear first, before you put pen to paper, about the overall structure it will have. *Planning* your essay makes all the difference between an essay which reads clearly, intelligently and smoothly, and one which is plain hard work to mark. I suggest that planning your essay actually makes your job of writing it a good deal easier – and more enjoyable.

Checking your essay

When the last full stop has been typed or written, it is tempting to throw the essay on one side, never to set eyes on it again until it returns to you from the marker. Such a practice is understandable, but risky.

Have a break from it at this stage, by all means. Leave the essay for a couple of days (providing you are not working right up to the time limit) so that when you do reread it, it will be relatively fresh and you will spot mistakes more easily.

If you have planned your essay properly, it is unlikely that major errors will have occurred. Coming to the essay fresh will enhance your appreciation of its structure and of the main thrust of its argument.

Questions to ask yourself include:

- Does the essay actually address the topic set?
  It is all too easy mentally to 'rewrite' a question to one that you prefer.
- Does the writing flow smoothly, or are there sudden 'jolts' between paragraphs?
- If there are illustrations or tables, do they complement the text and are they understandable? Does each figure have an explanatory caption?
- Are all the pages numbered?
- Is there a margin as required by the college regulations?

 SAVING SUCCESSIVE DRAFTS OF YOUR WORK

The benefits of using a word processor in writing fresh drafts are clear. Mistakes in spelling and grammar can be rectified, headings and subheadings redrafted, and paragraphs inserted or deleted. Fresh references can be included. By contrast, to rewrite an essay by hand, or with a typewriter, is a daunting and time consuming task.

However, after you have redrafted an essay, consider changing its 'File name' slightly so that both the fresh draft and the original version are stored on your disk(s). If you stick to the same file name, e.g. ESSAY4, the new draft that you save will write over the earlier draft. It may be useful for you to have on disk earlier drafts to reread, in case you want to insert material from them that you deleted in a later version. What you need is a file name that easily identifies each new draft. Thus for the fourth essay of your course, you might save its first draft using the file name ESSAY4.1. A subsequent draft will be saved using ESSAY4.2, and another as ESSAY4.3. All three versions of the same essay will be stored on your disk(s), the only disadvantage of this being that memory space on your disk(s) will be more quickly used up.

N o t e s

6 Writing a care study

Key topics

- Choosing a suitable patient or client for your care study
- Planning and setting out the care study
- Utilizing research-based care
- Problems commonly associated with writing a care study

Unlike examination questions, which are sometimes built around brief profiles of imaginary patients, the *care study* a student is required to write as part of the assessment strategy is based on an actual person – a patient or client for whom the student has cared. The fact that the subject of the study actually exists demands certain safeguards in its preparation and presentation. Of the many regulations set out by your college for your care study, perhaps the most important will concern the guarding of your patient's or client's well-being and confidentiality.

Safety first

Guarding the client's well-being

The client or patient on whom you base your care study will be chosen not only by you but also by your ward mentor (or your community supervisor) and perhaps also with the advice of your personal tutor.

A little later I'll discuss factors relating to the choice of client. Here I simply want to get across to you how important it is that, by choosing your client and by writing about her, you do her no harm. You may wonder how this could possibly occur. Indeed, it is the experience of many students that patients and clients are delighted to be chosen as the subject of a care study, and are only too willing to help.

There is, however, the possibility of harm being done, hence the importance of involving your mentor in your choice of client. A patient on your ward, for example, may not be fully aware of her diagnosis or of the results of tests. It is comparatively easy for a student to ask the patient during an interview a seemingly innocent question that reveals more than the student intends. 'Has the consultant from St Mary's been to see you yet?' may come as a shock to a patient who knows St Mary's as the hospital where people with cancer go for radiation treatment.

During an interview for a care study, it is almost inevitable (indeed, preferable) that a relationship builds between student and patient. After all, from the patient's point of view here is a nurse or therapist spending more time with her than almost anyone else has during her hospital stay. Within such a relationship, patients may feel able to ask questions they wouldn't have considered asking other busy professionals.

Interviews with clients are best planned rather than played by ear and, if you aren't used to conducting interviews, you may consider asking your mentor to attend your first few efforts. By planning an interview you stand a better chance of steering the patient away from *her* asking *you* embarrassing questions. If you have your

> **ACTIVITY**
>
> You are interviewing an elderly woman whose arthritic hip is giving her great pain. She suddenly fixes you with a beady eye and says, 'This old hip isn't going to get any better, is it? They'll have to operate, won't they?'
>
> Now, if you are a student nurse in your first year of training, you may feel that it isn't up to you to tell this patient what treatment is proposed for her. You may not be all that sure yourself. How might you or your colleagues deal with a situation like this?
>
> By telling her the first reassuring thing that comes into your head – 'Don't worry, I'm sure everything will be fine' – you may send out a message that you don't intend.

mentor close by he can quickly step in and retrieve a situation that looks like getting out of hand.

Guarding the client's confidentiality

Every patient has the right to confidential treatment. As a student physiotherapist, occupational therapist, or nurse, you will know that to chat about patients away from the clinical or educational area is a serious infringement of patients' rights. Patients can be identified from snippets of conversation overheard at the bus stop or in a pub.

Similarly, patients or clients may be identifiable from your care study. And care studies can be mislaid or left open on library tables while you hunt for a reference.

> Take all steps to avoid identifying your chosen client or patient.

Your college assessment regulations will require you to change your chosen patient's name. You should ensure this is done not only within the text of your study but also in any appendices – perhaps photocopies of hospital drug charts or fluid balance charts attached to the study folder to provide additional information. Check that such photocopies do not include the patient's real name, address, date of birth or hospital number, *anything* that may reveal his identity.

Sometimes changing the name isn't enough. You may be asked to provide some social background to your client, and often this is unlikely to provide any means of identification: 'Mrs Hemmel is 48 years old, married, with two young sons.'

But in other cases there may be a slight chance of revealing the patient's identity if certain details place him or her in a small or easily identifiable minority: 'David Lodge is a 36-year-old maths teacher at a local public school.' Or: 'Alison, 42, is the leader of a mountain rescue team in Derbyshire.'

You should make every effort to ensure that in no respect does your care study identify your chosen patient or client.

Choosing an appropriate client

Having dealt with the important 'safety' aspects of your study, we now turn to the broad guidelines that assist your choice of subject.

First of all, the patient must give his or her consent to be the subject of your care study. You should explain what 'care study' means, perhaps showing your patient one you've already written. You should assure your patient that he will not be identified from what you write, and that the study will be seen only by your teachers and assessors. You may also explain what are the steps involved in writing a care study, including reading your patient's medical and nursing notes, and interviewing him at least once. If he is a patient in hospital, you might also ask if you can visit him at home after his discharge, to see how well he is coping.

What sort of patient could you choose? Your assessment regulations might stipulate certain client characteristics for this particular assessment: a surgical patient, an elderly person living at home, or someone admitted to the acute ward of a mental health hospital.

Apart from these factors, however, there is a major consideration which will guide your choice of client or patient. He should demonstrate the vital interaction with your health care profession. What I mean is this: if you are a **student nurse**, the patient you choose should be the recipient of important (and interesting) nursing interventions. Your care study will concentrate on these nursing interventions rather than, say, any complex surgery he may have received.

As a **student physiotherapist**, you may choose for your care study a young man with ankylosing spondylitis (an arthritic condition of the spine). Perhaps you worked with him as a hospital patient receiving hydrotherapy. Your care study will show how beneficial exercising in warm water can be, how much his spinal movements improved and how you measured that improvement. Now he is about to go home and you devise a programme of joint and breathing exercises that he can take home with him. The emphasis of your care study will be on the role of the physiotherapist in the care of an individual, and so, of course, you choose a client for whom your role can readily be demonstrated.

As a **student occupational therapist**, you might choose an elderly patient recovering from a stroke on a medical ward. You work with him by helping him dress, teaching him how to use specially designed cutlery and kitchen gadgets. In short, your role is building up both his skills and his self-confidence and preparing him for discharge to, hopefully, his own home.

In these examples, the care studies will show how each of the students worked with other professionals, such as surgeons and physicians. The studies may also contain background information about the drugs prescribed for the patient, but each study will concentrate on the input from that particular health profession to which the student belongs.

> Your care study should emphasize the role of your chosen profession in caring for the client or patient.

Remember that you are writing a *care* study not a *case* study, which, to me, suggests something medically-based. If, as a student nurse, you choose a patient who has undergone surgery, a blow-by-blow account of the events inside the patient's abdomen is not what is needed. A succinct description of the operation is sufficient. Your study will concentrate on how you, as a nurse, managed the *care* of that *person*, not the management of a medical diagnosis.

Try and resist any temptation to choose a patient for the sake of his highly complex surgery. The obvious problem here is that you could get bogged down in unwanted surgical technicalities, leaving the poor patient uncared for, just the owner of a long list of '-ectomies'.

An important check list

As with any written assessment, there are certain factors about which you need to be absolutely clear before you begin even to plan your study. These factors were described in detail in Chapter 3 but here they are listed just as a reminder:

- **Title.** Is an exact title set, and are you allowed any choice within the title?
- **Word count.** Is there a single figure or a range? If the former, what discrepancy is allowable?
- **Submission date and time.** Note it in your diary, preceded by several 'early warning' entries.
- **Instructions regarding presentation.** How many copies are required, and what type of folder? Should the study be typed or may it be handwritten, and are

illustrations permitted?
- **References.** What reference system is required by your college? Is the client care you discuss to be based on research findings?
- **Marking scheme.** How are the marks awarded?
- Is a review of the client's **social background** required?
- Should your care study contain a **care plan** for your client or patient?
- If a nursing care study, should the patient care you discuss be based on a given **nursing model**, or on a model you may choose?

Using references for care

Your assessment regulations may stipulate that the care you discuss in your study should, wherever possible, be research-based. For example, in writing about the assessment of your patient for signs of pressure sore development you may refer to the literature relating to that particular assessment tool your ward used – Norton, Waterlow, or some other.

To help you in this, your ward may have a collection of relevant literature as a learning resource for its staff and students. The research studies contained within a ward folder shouldn't, of course, be considered as the sum of knowledge on your subject but as springboards to further items in the literature.

Visiting staff, from your own or other professions, may have useful references they can share with you and those references may in turn suggest others.

It would be unduly optimistic, however, to expect all clinical areas you come across, and all nursing care, to be founded on research. It might be that you find yourself on a ward where the ward manager and her staff firmly believe that pressure areas are best treated by being briskly rubbed with hospital spirit every 4 hours (to 'harden the skin' no doubt), or that every patient should be woken at 6 a.m. to have her temperature taken.

How you deal with such a situation, as a student challenging entrenched trained staff, lies outside the scope of this book. (You might well be advised to obtain the support of other students working with you, perhaps those senior to you, or the help of the ward's or your own tutor.) Your tact and your communication skills will be, to put it mildly, severely tested. However, the immediate problem is: how do you write a research-based care study when the care you are delivering is far from research-based?

My advice is not to lie. Don't describe care for your patient that simply hasn't been given. Instead, you can use your care study to point out – with gentle irony if you like – those areas of nursing or therapeutic care which are not founded on research but instead on myth, magic, and the decibel level of the manager's voice. Be careful not to be libellous: don't describe the ward manager as a brain-dead has-been, even if that is your private opinion. If you feel angry at the apparent deficiencies in care that you observe, and if your best efforts at protest come to nothing, you must turn your attention to looking after yourself: your self-esteem, your faith in yourself and your chosen profession. First of all, you can promise yourself that you'll never do the same when *you* are trained. Second, you can make use of your care study to relieve your frustration. It is amazing how much anger you can rid yourself of by 'writing it out.'

Telling it like it is

As I've already suggested, it is important that your care study describes accurately the care that is given to your chosen patient. It is perhaps superfluous further to point out that your chosen client should really exist.

The point of your care study is to show how you have planned and carried out the care for a certain individual. It is *not* a statement of how people with appendicitis are looked after, or youngsters with depression, or elderly people with pneumonia. My own college of health studies requires each student's ward or community mentor to sign the submitted care study, in order to show that it is the student's own work, and that the patient or client does exist.

Sometimes a student's language gives the game away. The care study starts soundly enough but then lapses occur. I find myself reading: 'The patient should be prepared for theatre by asking her to remove her dentures, if she has any, and by . . .' This isn't the care study of a real patient; this is an instructional manual for patients having an operation. Compare the sentence above with the following:

■ *'Mrs Cambridge was asked if she wore dentures. I explained that they had to be removed before her operation in order to assist the anaesthetist . . .'*

Can you see the difference? The second sentence certainly seems to be describing *care that has actually been given*. In this respect, I find care studies one of the most valuable of the assessment tools available to health care courses (and far more valuable, I believe, than unseen exams).

Organizing the care study

The scope of the care study may be set out for you in your college's assessment regulations. These might stipulate that the patient's social background must be described, or her psychological state, as well as her physical and physiological condition. You may be asked to describe the relevance of the tests she undergoes, and to explain the altered physiology relating to her medical condition. You should carefully follow such requirements.

I put forward the following suggested outline for a care study for you to consider. Bear in mind that how you organize your own study will very much depend on the health care course you are taking as well as the patient or client you've chosen.

- Introduction – fictitious name of client, age, and family background.
- Other social details, such as employment, area where she lives, and type of dwelling.
- The setting in which you provided care – hospital, hospice, industry, client's own home.
- Medical, nursing or therapeutic reason for care being delivered. (For example, the client is unable to cope with cooking for himself after the death of his wife and his current episode of depression.)
- Client's own understanding of reasons for admission or visit.
- Any relevant medical history. (Be very careful as you work your way through pages of medical notes on your patient. A hernia operation 27 years ago won't be very relevant to a patient's current admission for depression; but if a 6-year-old child is admitted to a ward for removal of his tonsils, a previous hospital stay – and his reaction to that experience – would be highly important.)
- Relevant altered physiology. An elderly man with a hernia, for example, might lead you to demonstrate your understanding of the condition, perhaps by drawing a diagram of the normal small intestine, followed by one showing an inguinal hernia. You could then discuss the possible complications that can arise from herniation. As a general rule you should show the links between normal human physiology and how it changes in disease or trauma.
- Medical tests being performed – brief description and explanation. Give your

patient's results (for example, of the blood tests she has had) together with the normal values for those tests.

- Care delivered to your patient or client. This may be for a single day or for some other period of time, as specified by your assessment regulations: perhaps the period following operation or leading to the patient's discharge. Your patient is first *assessed*, possibly by yourself and your mentor. Relatives might be involved in this process. You should show how care is *planned* and how your client was involved (if appropriate) in the planning of his own care. The objectives of care should be demonstrably achievable within a stated timespan. Your discussion should then cover the *delivery* of the planned care, perhaps showing how other professionals were involved. You should then show how your care was *evaluated* and, perhaps, altered.

    (What I have briefly described above is the *process* of nursing, a systematic method of managing and delivering *individualized care* that is equally appropriate for medicine and remedial therapy. For student nurses presently unfamiliar with the nursing process, you could read Kenworthy et al (1995) as a sound introduction. For a more detailed discussion see Chapter 5 in Roper et al (1990). It is a subject, however, that will be covered in depth throughout your nursing course.)

- The course of your client's condition following the period you are discussing – discharge to his own home, transfer to a hospice, or perhaps death. (Don't regard a patient's death as a failure of nursing or therapeutic care, and as such not suitable for your care study. You might like to consider how successful care can contribute to a peaceful and dignified death, in which the patient's needs, and those of his relatives, are met.)
- References.
- Bibliography (if required).
- Appendices, for example photocopied drug charts or observation charts. The earlier warning is repeated here – ensure there is nothing on these that will identify your patient or client.

The patient profile outlined in the following activity box is provided for your consideration and discussion with your colleagues. It is a longer profile than those previously found in this text. It concerns a young woman who, following a miscarriage and separation from her boyfriend, takes an overdose of her antidepressant tablets.

Here are some suggested points of especial interest:

- Sally's social background
- the causes of her overdose
- the importance of observations
- how to encourage Sally to carry out breathing exercises
- how to get through to such a withdrawn person
- the risk of Sally harming herself – how should she be observed during her stay on your ward? (For example, should she be nursed in a single room, for privacy and quiet, or in a large bay for ease of observation? This is a tricky point.)
- who should care for her? It is usually easy to arrange for female nurses and therapists to carry out Sally's care; but at what stage might male staff be introduced to her? Could this be used as a means of helping Sally view men as caring and compassionate, following her disastrous experience?

Now here are two suggested danger areas:

- The emergency treatment in Accident Service. This would be useful background material but, unless your care study is specifically set in this department, you shouldn't dwell on the intricacies of emergency care and management.
- The risk of cardiac arrhythmias and the observation of Sally's cardiac monitor. An overdosage of an antidepressant drug like amitriptyline can lead to cardiac

ACTIVITY – A PATIENT TRANSFER

Claire, a staff nurse from the Accident Ward, has accompanied Sally, the patient, to your ward. While two nurses help Sally into bed, Claire gives the ward manager and yourself a summary of the patient and her care while in her charge. As you listen to the staff nurse, you wonder whether Sally would be a good patient for your care study. (I've tried to devise Sally's profile so that it will be of interest to you as a student physiotherapist, occupational therapist, or nurse.)

As you read what follows, note which parts of the report could be useful for your care study, and which parts might be danger signals: those topics where you could get too involved in detail which isn't vital for your care study.

■ 'Thank you for taking this patient, sister. Her name is Sally Henderson, and she's 31 years old. She is unmarried but she's had the same boyfriend for the past 4 years – until recently, that is.'

'A couple of months ago she discovered she was pregnant – she'd been living with her boyfriend for some time – and she felt that he wasn't too happy about it. However, a week ago she had a miscarriage. When she told Peter, the boyfriend, he packed his bags and left her. They didn't have a row – he just left.'

'She was extremely upset. She felt she couldn't tell her parents because they'd never liked Peter, and now they'd been proved right. She'd been given amitriptyline tablets 50 mg twice a day by her GP, and two days ago she took the lot – probably about 25 tablets in all.'

'Luckily, just after she did this, Peter came back to fetch some records he'd forgotten. He found her practically unconscious and phoned for an ambulance. He waited for the ambulance to arrive, and then cleared off again.'

'Sally had a stomach washout in Accident Service, and we sent the contents off to Path Lab for analysis. Naturally, we had Sally on a cardiac monitor in case of arrhythmias, but she's been in sinus rhythm ever since. However, the consultant wants her to stay on a monitor while she's on the general ward – just in case.'

'What else is there to tell you . . . ? She's hardly taken anything to eat or drink, and she appears very, very withdrawn. She doesn't look at you while you speak to her, just stares at the wall.'

'Her parents have visited – very upset, of course, why didn't she tell us, that sort of thing. But they seem very supportive, and they'll visit regularly, I'm sure. We've asked them not to confront Sally about the overdose but just to chat about ordinary things at home for the time being.'

'Observations – well, there's the heart monitor. The consultant wants hourly pulse, 2-hourly blood pressure, and 4-hourly temperature. Chest physiotherapy has to be carried out every 4 hours – I forgot to mention that she inhaled some vomit before she got to Accident Service, and part of her lung is affected. Try and get her to cough and to breathe deeply.'

'You'll need to keep a close eye on her, that's for sure. The doctor reckons she's still a bad suicide risk. I just wish we could get through to her, somehow . . .'

'Oh, one more thing. Charles, our ward manager, went to her yesterday to do her blood pressure and she got very upset indeed. So at the moment we have just female nurses looking after her. I think she reckons all men are stinkers – she could well be right!'

After reading this handover report from Claire, discuss with your colleagues the most interesting points you've noticed. Which aspects of Sally's care – whether nursing or therapy – do you think could prove most interesting to discuss in your care study based on Sally? And which are the 'danger points' – areas where it would be all too easy to become entangled with overtechnical detail?

Once you've done this, try drawing up a plan – perhaps using headings and subheadings as I suggested in an earlier chapter – for Sally's care study.

arrhythmias (unusual and sometimes dangerous rhythms of the heartbeat). The student could get too involved with the various possible heart rhythms observed on the cardiac monitor. This would be appropriate for, say, a care study based on one of the coronary care unit (CCU) patients. A brief mention of perhaps the most dangerous of the arrhythmias for which nurses must observe is perhaps all that is needed for a care study based on a patient on a general medial ward. Remember that you are writing a care study about a *person* – not a machine.

In your discussion with colleagues, you may well come up with more danger points or areas of especial interest.

Avoiding value judgements

Claire, the staff nurse in the above patient profile, made one or two value judgements in her handover – the main one being an aside about the male of the species. Perhaps her comment was justified in its context? However, in discussing the care of your chosen patient or client it is wiser to avoid making value judgements – criticisms, either overt or covert, about the subject of your study. (This is something you should certainly do when you come to write nursing notes on a care plan.)

Here are two examples of the type of value statements I mean:

- *Mr James seemed to have a low pain threshold.*
- *Mrs Wilks frequently demanded attention by pressing her call button.*

Neither of these is particularly damaging, but both express the carer's opinion of the client. The term 'low pain threshold' could be regarded as a statement of fact, but it can, from my nursing experience, be used dismissively:

- *'He's got a low pain threshold – he doesn't really need another injection.'*
  (If you think about this, a patient with a low pain threshold surely needs a pain killer.)

In the second statement, the frequency with which Mrs Wilks presses her call button may well be a matter of fact – but the use of the word 'demanded' adds a judgemental factor.

Neither of these two statements should appear in a care study. What *is* both relevant and interesting, however, is your reaction to your chosen client, as his professional carer. If you are irritated by your client, if you simply don't like him, you may well wish to discuss this in your study. (You may, of course, feel it is better to choose another client.) What exactly is it about the client's personality or behaviour that angers you? And how do you try and care for him pleasantly and effectively? What measures do you take to overcome your feelings? Did other members of the health care team feel the same as you? All these questions are worth discussing, because they may give you insights into your own character as well as that of your client.

Incorporating a care plan within the care study

With the importance of individualized care stressed in your health care course, the patients or clients you care for will have care plans on which their daily care is based. These care plans may reflect the model of care (such as the Roper, Logan and Tierney model of nursing) that is used on a ward or within a community team. Read your assessment regulations to discover whether your care *study* should incoporate a care *plan*.

I would make two points about care plans:

1. Each care plan emphasizes that the client is an individual, with his own problems and needs and, therefore, his individual nursing or therapeutic interventions. No longer do we learn about 'the care of a hernia' or 'looking after a heart attack' in our colleges of health. Instead, we learn about assessing an individual's problems in order to plan and implement care that is geared towards solving those problems.
2. Care plans should *direct the care*. Used properly, care plans are not pieces of paper which, annoyingly, have to be filled in at the end of a busy shift – as a summary of what's been done for the client. It is to the care plan that a patient's nurse turns at the beginning of her shift in order to discover what care is required by him that day. If a patient's named nurse, or primary nurse (see Kenworthy et al 1995) is ill, or on holiday, another nurse should be able to pick up the care plan and continue with the planned care.

In the next chapter I discuss the challenges of searching the literature (for example, making use of libraries), using references, and writing a literature review.

REFERENCES
Kenworthy N Concepts of individual care. In: Kenworthy N, Snowley G, Gilling C 1992 Common foundation studies in nursing. Churchill Livingstone, Edinburgh
Roper N, Logan W W, Tierney A J 1990 The elements of nursing , 3rd edn. Churchill Livingstone, Edinburgh

Notes

7 Searching and reviewing the literature

Key topics

■ Using libraries and catalogues
■ Writing references to the literature
■ Writing a critical literature review

Earlier in the book I briefly mentioned one reason for including in your essay or project references to the literature: that of backing up a statement you want to make (see pp. 22–23). When you write something for a college assessment, or for submitting to a professional journal for publication, you are far more careful about making assertions than you might be if your were arguing with friends in a pub. To your friends you might feel able to say, 'Students these days are far lazier than when I did my course.' What you are sharing in this conversation is an opinion, perhaps based on unsystematic observation or on hearsay. You are *not* stating a proven fact.

To back up such a statement in an essay, however, you would need to refer to an educational researcher who had carried out a study on students over the past 10 or more years. (You would also need to express your view somewhat more carefully.)

Referring to the literature in your essay or project serves another purpose. It shows the assessor that you have studied the background to your subject, that you have sifted through what has already been written about it, have analysed it as best you can, and can present your findings in a concise and logical manner.

A review of the literature can also serve to 'fine-tune' your choice of subject for a research project: what has already been written will push you away from one aspect of your chosen subject and point you in the direction of another. It will help you to choose one research tool (such as a questionnaire) and to reject another (interviews). One particular piece of literature may suggest that it would be suitable for replication – for repeating, but in today's social climate rather than that in which it was originally written. Another study may sound appealing, but on closer reading you discover the writer makes his assertions from a study with only four student nurses as his research material. You decide that this makes his assertions decidedly suspect and you want to carry out your own study, but with 24 student nurse subjects.

You will already have realized that a review of the literature, when incorporated into your research study or special project, is far more than a string of names and dates. Writing a literature review can be a useful assessment for health care students in its own right, for it encourages students to read carefully and critically, and to put together a logical summary of what they've read.

There is, too, a practical value to carrying out a literature review, since it encourages students to get to grips with their college library. It persuades them to prowl the shelves they haven't previously looked at, to examine banks of card catalogues, and even to try out that computerized catalogue they've so far been too scared to touch. It also suggests sources of information other than the library attached to their own college.

Searching the literature

Getting to know the librarian

Put from your mind all stereotypical images of librarians as fierce ladies whose job it is to date-stamp your books and to 'shush' you if you so much as cough inside their hallowed halls.

Librarians are best regarded as managers of information. They may not have at their fingertips facts about, say, parenteral nutrition, but they can certainly tell you where to find them. Librarians are experts for their own library: its individual system of classifying books and journals, the specialist collections it houses, and its various catalogues.

They participate in 'networks': formal or informal links with librarians in their own and other specialist fields, in other parts of the country, and in other countries. Librarians are thus able to tap into the specialist knowledge of many sources of information.

Tours of the college library can be arranged through its staff, tours which take in the arrangement of its books, how the professional journals are held, and the existence of special collections. (These are sometimes bequeathed to libraries from former members of the college staff who don't want to see their collection (both books and journals) split up, since its main value lies in its being held together. Such collections may be held in different buildings, or in locked cupboards, so that the new student may be unaware of their existence.)

Librarians can refer students to members of staff with certain areas of interest. For example, a student in my own college became very keen on working with disabled people in Afghanistan, having seen a television programme about the huge numbers of people there with legs blown off by land mines. There was little about disability in the college library, but the librarian put the student in touch with me. My interest in disability issues had led me to form a large collection of disability books, reports and articles, together with my own catalogue. The librarian served as the vital link between student and specialist information source.

 WRITING FOR PUBLICATION

All I have written so far about librarians is relevant to authors researching areas of particular interest. It is common for writers to speak highly of the librarians in their local towns and in those parts of the world they visit. It is my own experience that librarians are genuinely pleased to be asked to help a writer, often entering into the spirit of a search that can be long, tiring, but never tedious.

The best general rule is: if you're stuck with a project, if your search of the shelves has proved fruitless, then *ask for help*. Librarians are a tremendous source of both information and encouragement. They are one of the best learning resources within a college.

Making effective use of your college library

Don't wait until a specific job takes you to your library, such as hunting for a certain book or looking up a reference. Make the time at the beginning of your course to walk leisurely around the library. Glance along its shelves to get some idea of how the books are ordered and the shelves labelled. Look into odd corners where there might be shelves of books or journals partly hidden out of the way. Note which books may be loaned and which are for reference purposes only.

Find out whether your library has a 'stack'. This is a collection of specialist material – both books and journals – held in a different part of the library, sometimes in a basement area. The stack I used when at university consisted of huge metal shelves which were moved along 'railway lines' by an electric motor. There were so many shelves in the stack they were too close together for the researcher to get in between, unless he first moved apart the ones he wanted to use along the lines. (You had to make sure there was no silent student further along the stack, in case he got squashed when you moved your shelves.)

You need to discover whether there is a quiet area of the library for private study, and what the times are for the library to open and close. You should find out how long books may be kept on loan, and what the procedure is for renewing any books you need to keep longer. There will be a system for requesting books, and also for ordering photocopies of articles from journals not held by your own college library.

Many libraries now use a computerized catalogue and bibliography. The latter can be held on a CD (compact disk) and is referred to as a CD-ROM (Read Only Memory: this means that you can't add anything to the memory stored on the compact disk, or alter it in any way). This CD-based bibliography is excellent for holding huge amounts of information. You may well find references for articles and pieces of research in languages other than English. However, sometimes an abstract (a brief summary) is available in English and can be both read from the screen and printed on paper.

Looking through the shelves of journals, you may find that some – like *Nursing Times* and *Nursing Standard* – include very brief summaries each week of the latest relevant medical, nursing and social research. Such reviews are a good means of keeping in touch with research that is published in areas other than the one in which you're presently interested.

You'll also discover that some journals are more immediately approachable, more reader-friendly, than others. I don't think it is doing *Nurse Education Today* a disservice to suggest that its articles are somewhat more taxing to read and understand than many of those in the weekly journals mentioned above.

Sometimes, however, you'll find that a piece of research can be reported in detail in one journal, while a shorter and simpler version is issued in another. A report in the *British Medical Journal*, for example, can appear, greatly simplified, in *Nursing Standard's* research précis page.

Using other sources of information

When hunting for books and articles on a certain subject, *be creative*. Don't confine yourself to your own college library, excellent though that may be. Its librarians will be the first to suggest that you look further afield. For matters on social policy, sociology or psychology, for example, it may be that the nearest big public library will have more information. It will certainly keep national and local newspapers, and their back copies, which may contain useful articles.

Universities and colleges of higher and further education may also make their libraries available to health care students, especially if there are formal links with the health college. Hospitals with medical schools will have excellent libraries, but other district hospitals may well have libraries attached to their postgraduate medical centres.

It may be that the topic you have been set for your written assessment has particular relevance to local groups, including pressure groups. For example, a subject like 'Problems of communication with patients and clients' may lead you not just to a shelf in your own library, but also to local centres for deaf and blind people. Here you will find pamphlets explaining the particular communication problems faced by these important client groups.

If you are researching the topic 'Dental provision in the community' you may come across a local Access Group which will have information on how many (or, more likely, how few) dental surgeries are accessible to people using wheelchairs or other walking aids.

> In searching for information, don't be static . . . look around and be creative!

By sticking to the one familiar college library, you really are restricting the amount of information that is available to you for your research, essay or project. Set out on a voyage of exploration, and see what you can discover!

Searching the literature is rather like the detective work in those crime novels enjoyed by most of us – one clue turns up, and it leads to another, and then to another. So it is with references to the literature. The first article you find is excellent in itself, but its importance lies also in its reference to other works, and these set you off in another direction (see Fig.7.1). The problem then is knowing when to stop. Usually it's time – or lack of it – that forces you to stop searching, to examine what you've already obtained, and to write your literature review.

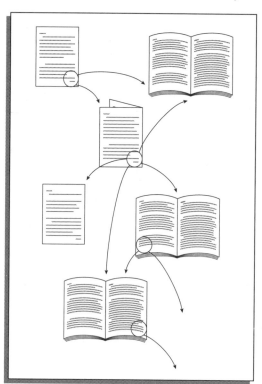

Figure 7.1
Searching for 'clues' in the literature.

Writing references to the literature

In the final section of this chapter, I discuss how to write a critical review of the literature. This section, however, deals with the technicalities of writing references – how to set out, both within your main text and at its end, in the Reference section, the important details of each item of the literature you've utilized.

There's one point I'd make first about writing references: they should be sufficiently full and accurate to enable your readers to seek out the literature to which you refer for themselves. This applies whichever system of referencing you choose to use (or whichever is required by your college or publisher).

WRITING FOR PUBLICATION

If you are preparing a manuscript for submission to a professional journal, you should ensure you use the system of referencing preferred by that journal. The same applies to manuscripts prepared for a publisher. Churchill Livingstone, for example, supplies its authors with guidance for writing references in its own preferred 'house style', and other publishers will do likewise.

You should note that, as an author, *you* are responsible for the accuracy of the references you include. It is not the job of your editor to check these for you.

In this section, I'm going to describe two methods of writing references to the literature – one which lists items in numerical order and one which lists items alphabetically. You should note, however, that there are variations within these two types.

Listing references numerically

With this method, the literature is referred to in your text by means of either a number in brackets, like this (1); or by a *superscript* number: that is, a number which is printed slightly above the line of type, like this[2]. If your word processor can't write superscript numbers (of if you're not sure how to do it) it is perfectly adequate to write your reference numbers in brackets. Once you've chosen which to do, though, be consistent. As you progress through your essay or project, new references are simply added numerically, like this[3]. If you want to refer to two or more items from the literature at the same point in your text, you simply separate the superscript or bracketed numbers by commas, thus[4,5,6]. Referring to a previously used item, you can write the number by which it was originally denoted[1] rather than giving it a new number[7].

In the reference section at the end of your study, the items of the literature are listed in their numerical order. The following are examples of references to books, to articles in journals, and to chapters within a multi-author book. I have made up titles, authors and publishers.

Reference to a book:

■ 1 Brown N. *Writing for publication.* London, Prima Books. 1992.

- author's surname and initial
- book's title, either underlined or printed in italics
- place of publication
- name of publisher
- year of publication

Reference to an article in a journal:

■ 2 Smith J. How to write an article. *Nursing Weekly* 1991, 4, 36, 55–57.

- author's surname and initial
- title of the article (some journals may require this title to be placed between inverted commas: '. . .')
- name of the journal either underlined or printed in italics
- year of publication
- volume of journal
- number of issue within the volume
- page number(s) of the article

Reference to a chapter or contribution to a multi-author book:

■ Black K Writing a scientific report. In: White L *Science and medicine.* Newcastle, Boffin Publications. 1990.

- chapter author's surname and initial
- title of chapter or contribution
- the word 'In' denoting following reference to main text
- author or editor of overall book
- name of book underlined or in italics
- place of publication
- name of publisher
- year of publication

If L White, of the above reference, was the book's editor, the following would occur after his name within brackets: (ed).

What happens when a book is written by, or edited by, more than one person? For two authors, both names can be mentioned within your study's main text:

■ As White and Brown state, writing for publication is a highly competitive business (8).

The full reference at the end of your study will provide both surnames and their initials.

For three or more authors, only the first author's surname need be mentioned in your text, but it is followed by the words *et al.* meaning 'and others'. Thus:

■ As White *et al.* remark, writing for publication does not make the author a rich person (9).

The full reference at the end of your study should include the names of *all* its authors even, I'm afraid, if there are many of them (as there can be with some scientific papers).

All this appears very complicated, doesn't it? However, what this system achieves is to provide your study with full and accurate references in a systematic and consistent way.

Having said that, I don't like this numerical system of listing references, though I have no choice but to use it when I'm writing for the two principal weekly nursing journals. Suppose you're almost through writing your study and you've so far listed 17 references. Suddenly, you realize that there is another reference to the literature that really ought to be included – but it comes in between your present references 3 and 4. This means that all the reference numbers from 4 onwards have to be changed. This problem doesn't occur with the author-based method I'm going to describe next.

Listing references alphabetically

A frequently used method of referencing is one called the Harvard system (presumably after the American university of that name), in which references are listed alphabetically by author and year of publication. Numbers in brackets or superscript numbers are not used within your text. Instead you'll find an author's surname, together with the year in which her book or article was published, as in the following example:

■ *Writing for publication is a difficult business, especially during a recession (Brown, 1992). Furthermore, it fails to raise much money for the hard-working author (White et al. 1991).*

In the final Reference section, the literature is listed in alphabetical order by authors' surnames. Where one author has two or more works listed, they appear in order of their years of publication, thus:

Black, A (1990)
Brown, T (1991)
Brown, T (1995)
Green, G (1987)
and so on.

Figures 7.2, 7.3 and 7.4 show different applications of the Harvard system, as references to the literature might appear in a card index system drawn up by a student. From these cards you can devise how references would appear in your project's final References and Bibliography sections.

Edwards, R & Williams, M (1989)
Caring for the anxious patient:
the role of the occupational
therapist.
Glasgow, Worldwide Press plc.

Figure 7.2
A reference to a book using the Harvard system of referencing.

Gregson, C.A. (1988)
'The arthritic client in the
community.'
Health and Social Professional,
4, 29, 70-72.

Figure 7.3
A reference to an article in a journal, using the Harvard system of referencing.

Meadows, C. (1991)
'Chest physiotherapy for the child
in intensive care.'
In
Anderson, B, Fletcher, N, &
Meadows, C (eds),
Paediatric critical care.
Newcastle, Prestige Press.

Figure 7.4
A reference to a contribution in a multi-author book using the Harvard system of referencing.

Figure 7.2 shows how a reference to a book is listed:

- surnames of the authors, with their respective initials
- year of publication in brackets
- title of book, either underlined or printed in italics
- place of publication
- name of publisher.

Figure 7.3 shows how a reference to an article in a journal is listed:

- surname of author, followed by initial(s)
- year of publication in brackets
- title of article enclosed in inverted commas
- title of journal, either underlined or printed in italics
- volume number of journal
- issue number within the volume
- page number(s) of article.

Figure 7.4 shows how a reference to a chapter in a multi-author book is listed:

- surname of chapter author, followed by initial(s)
- year of publication in brackets
- title of chapter or contribution enclosed in inverted commas
- the word 'In' denoting following reference to main text
- surnames of authors, followed by respective initial(s) – (ed) or (eds) denotes editorship of the book
- title of book, either underlined or printed in italics
- place of publication
- name of publisher.

Note how, in the case of a book, its title is underlined or printed in italics, whereas if the reference is to an article, the title of the journal appears underlined or in italics.

I would add one brief point about storing references to articles contained in journals. You will have noticed how the references in the above examples included journal volume and number, rather than the full date of publication (e.g. day and month, as well as year). This seems to be the usual practice, but you may find it useful to make a note on your own record cards of the full date of certain articles, especially if this will help you find them again in your college library.

If I'm given the choice, my preference is certainly for the Harvard system of referencing rather than the numerical system. One reason for this preference is that, when reading a text, I am likelier to recognize the source of a given reference from the author's surname rather than from a superscript or bracketted number. It is far easier, also, when reading through a draft of an article or essay, to fit in additional references – you don't have to alter numbers.

WRITING FOR PUBLICATION

Different publishers have different house styles covering minutiae such as where commas or semicolons are used, or whether the year of publication is written inside brackets. If you are writing for publication, you must follow your publisher's house style exactly. Similarly, if your college assessment information provides examples of referencing methods it prefers, stick to them.

If you glance through this book, you'll discover Churchill Livingstone's preferred house style of referencing (called the Ciba system). Is it based on the Harvard system or on the numerical system?

That's an easy question. But you'll also have noticed that the Churchill Livingstone style differs slightly from the examples given in Figures 7.2, 7.3 and 7.4, in that underlining, italics and brackets are not used. Also, the name of the publisher is placed before the place of publication – which I think is logical. The whole effect is somehow 'cleaner' and less fussy. Note also that some house styles of referencing require only the first word of a book title to begin with a capital letter, the rest being lower case. Other styles would begin most words of a title with a capital letter (except for 'a' or 'an' or 'the').

Quoting from the literature

It sometimes happens that an author to whom you wish to refer puts her argument in a way that you feel can neither be bettered nor shortened. In such an instance, you could consider quoting her, but here are three important guidelines about quoting from the literature.

First, remember that the assessment you're writing is supposed to be *your* work – not the author's. Quotations of 10 or 12 lines of text are simply too long. I'm not sure where the limit is – whether three lines of quotation are permissible but four lines aren't. You will have to judge this for yourself, or seek advice from your tutor. As a general rule, where you can paraphrase in order to state the crux of your author's argument succinctly, you should do so.

My second guideline is that you must quote accurately, even down to the punctuation. If you want to shorten a quotation, however, you can join together a couple of phrases that lie apart within the original text, by using three dots (called an ellipsis), as in the following examples. First, here is the text you want to quote, but you think it's too long:

■ *'In all his writing – his books, his articles, his short stories, and even his occasional broadcasts – Jones proved himself a master of the language.'*

Here is one way you could shorten it:

■ *'In all his writing . . . Jones proved himself a master of the language'* (Simon 1990, p. 50).

And here is another. Perhaps in your essay you've mentioned the name 'Jones' rather too close to the quote you want to make. How can you quote this passage yet omit the name?

■ *'In all his writing . . .(he) proved himself a master of the language'* (Simon 1990, p. 50).

Here you've inserted a word so that your quote makes grammatical sense (and remains accurate), but to show that 'he' is your word, not the author's, you've enclosed it in brackets.

The third guideline is that the page number of the quoted reference should be included, as shown in these examples. Where you refer to a book or article in a general way, rather than to a specific sentence or passage, no page number is needed.

Does all this sound complicated and confusing? It really is necessary, however, to provide *accurate* references in a consistent way. Unfortunately mistakes occur, even in books and articles that are published, and these can mislead the reader. In a highly respected book on disability, I found a reference to the literature that sounded very exciting:

■ *'Screaming Stereotypes: Images of Disabled People in Television and the Motion Pictures.'*

Following up this reference I discovered its real title was somewhat less exciting: 'Screening Stereotypes . . .'

To repeat: references to and quotations from the literature should be *accurate*.

Writing a critical literature review

The previous section of this chapter has dealt with the fairly mechanical matter of writing references accurately – where to put the brackets, what to underline, and so on. Once you get into the habit of writing your references in the manner required by your college (or publisher) it will become easier.

This section, however, is the 'meat' of the chapter, for it concerns the nature of the literature review that you intend to write. It has occasionally seemed to me, in marking students' assessments, that they are unaware of the reasons for including a review of the literature within a project. Instead, perhaps through glancing at reviews in published studies, they have wrongly formed the conclusion that a literature review is simply a list of names and dates. They assume that the more references their review includes, the more marks they will gain. This is definitely not the case.

Let me try and demonstrate what I mean. Read through the following mock literature review, in which I've incorporated imaginary references. What do you make of it?

■ *Brown 1990 states that nurses' assessment of the surgical patient's pain is inadequate. White 1991 bears this out, her research showing that nurses almost always underestimated the pain experienced by postoperative patients. Some further research by Black 1992 showed that pain assessment by nurses was closer to that made by house surgeons rather than the amount of pain claimed by their postoperative patients.*

Well, at least my literature review has squeezed in three references! How many marks do you think I deserve for that?

> A literature review is more than a list of names and dates.

My view is: not many. All this review demonstrates is that X says this, Y says that, and Z says the other. It is neither detailed nor critical. An assessor would be justified in asking whether I had *really* read what Brown, White and Black had found. Neither have I shown I understand the methodologies chosen for their research by each writer, nor my understanding of any doubtful claims they might have made.

Most important, I have shown no links between these references and the study in which I'm currently engaged. For example, have these three studies caused me to change my approach to my own study, to utilize a particular research tool in preference to another? Perhaps I'm not engaged in writing a research study, but rather a large-scale project on postoperative pain control for which a literature review is required by my college. Even here, I must show that I can *critically* assess the literature to which I refer. Perhaps the literature I've discovered shows me that my project ought to include a section on Pain Clinics – something I'd not previously thought about. Perhaps the literature mentions means of controlling pain other than using drugs, and this again suggests a further section to my project – or else it suggests I devote my entire project to a narrower subject, such as alternative methods of pain control. Whatever the case, I have to show there is some degree of interaction between my study and the literature I discuss.

A literature review is not a shopping list. It is not a salt and pepper addition to a study, sprinkled liberally over the pages: the more salt and pepper I sprinkle, the more marks I get.

Let me now rework part of the above example of a literature review, and try and show the type of discussion that might be included. Again, the reference is imaginary.

■ *Initially, the findings of Brown 1990 convinced me that my choice of project subject was sound: how well nurses assess their patients' pain. Brown's research seemed to suggest that nurses' assessment of the pain experienced by surgical patients was almost always underestimated. Closer examination of her study, however, revealed that it took place on two surgical wards, all of whose patients were under the care of the same consultant surgeon and anaesthetist. One staff nurse interviewed by Brown makes the important point that since, in her view, the patients were written up for inadequate analgesia, nurses were not encouraged to assess their patients' pain accurately. There was little point, the nurse said, in discovering the level of a patient's pain, if you were unable then to relieve it effectively (Brown 1990, pp. 31–32). Brown seems to have ignored this nurse's views in her conclusions. Could it be that the nurses in Brown's study sought to protect themselves by underestimating their patients' pain?*

Only one reference here – but there is a much deeper discussion about that one piece of research. An important shortcoming in the study's design is highlighted, as is the relationship between that study and the student's own project. Originally he was well satisfied with his choice of project subject – now he's having second thoughts. His literature review might go on to show how, by reading more studies, he intends to 'slant' his project topic to include an examination of how effectively prescribed analgesia is actually given by surgical ward nurses.

Of course, your literature review may also confirm you in your choice of project topic. To review 'critically' does not mean you are obliged to pick holes in the literature. You are allowed to praise it, too.

As a general rule, I would rather see somewhat fewer references sprinkled throughout the pages of a literature review and more in the way of a general discussion. However, I'm not prepared to suggest a 'correct' number of references you might need and I doubt if your tutor will either.

One of the RCN studies that does not contain a discrete literature review (that is, one labelled as such) is Atkinson & Sklaroff 1987, a study dealing with the care of physically disabled people admitted to acute hospital wards. The research itself, however, seems to have grown out of one nursing paper, published some years

> **ACTIVITY**
>
> As a brief activity, have another look at my reworked review above. You will see how I've used the first person pronouns, 'me' and 'my'. Perhaps you remember the discussion in Chapter 4 about the use of the so-called 'academic style'. Can you think of any advantage in the above review to using the first person pronouns? How do you think it reads? Do you think 'the writer' or 'the present writer' would have been an improvement?
>
> Note too the occasion in the review where I incorporated an exact reference to the imaginary researcher Brown, including a page number. Why was this necessary at that point?
>
> You may wish now to look through some of the Royal College of Nursing (RCN) research papers, concentrating on how each author has written her or his review of the literature. Concentrate on how the literature is discussed (rather than listed), how links are formed between some of the references given, and between certain references and the author's present study. Your college library may also keep copies in its reference section of students' past projects (usually those of a high quality). By reading these, you can see how your predecessors have coped with writing a good, in-depth, critical review of the literature.

before (Blackwood 1978); it could be said that Blackwood 1978 inspired the later research.

It does seem strange to me, though, for such an important study *not* to include a thorough literature review. One of my criticisms of Atkinson & Sklaroff 1987 is that their investigation places disability firmly within the medical model (with disability perceived as arising from a medical diagnosis). Had the authors consulted disability literature – including that written by disabled authors – they might have discovered that their view of disability was out of date. In my opinion, they failed to allow their prior assumptions about disability to be challenged by the disability literature.

The preceding paragraph, which in itself is an example (good or bad) of a mini literature review, concludes this chapter. Chapter 8 discusses the particular problems associated with writing a large-scale project, and handling large amounts of information.

REFERENCES
Atkinson F I , Sklaroff S A 1987 Acute hospital wards and the disabled patient: a survey of the experiences of patients and nurses. Royal College of Nursing, London
Blackwood M 1978 Disability without handicap: a cry from the heart. Nursing Times 74 (33): 22–23 (Supplement)

N o t e s

8 Writing a large-scale project

Key topics

■ Planning a large-scale project
■ Storing a large amount of information
■ Retrieving information required for your project

Although the sort of project discussed here is not a research study (for which I would recommend Bell 1987 as a guide) it may well require you to engage in some of the activities necessary in conducting research. In planning your project, for example, you will certainly have to undertake a literature search in order to amass information, and probably write a literature review.

It is this gathering of information which, I think, presents students with some of their greatest problems in writing a large-scale piece of work – both collecting it in the initial stages, and then reassembling it as they plan and write their project. In brief, the information they gather has to be readily retrievable, and this is discussed in a later section of this chapter. Another problem, to be discussed shortly, is that of setting the boundaries of your study – establishing a subject which is tightly enough defined to provide you with sufficient 'meat' for your project while preventing you overrunning your word count. I'll be giving examples of such boundaries later.

You may find useful the earlier discussions in Chapters 4 and 5 on presentation and structure in an essay. The sort of project I have in mind for this present chapter is about three times the length of an essay (depending, of course, on your college's assessment requirements); it is perhaps true to say that achieving a clear structure is more important the longer the piece of work being planned. In a project, you may choose to use a series of sections (you could even call them chapters) with explanatory titles, as well as incorporating headings and subheadings within each of these sections. Just as you should be consistent in the printed appearance of your headings (using bold, underlining, or italic script, or even differing type sizes), so you should with your section or chapter titles.

An important check list

Meanwhile here is a reminder of the information it is important for you to have at your fingertips while planning your project. For earlier discussion of each of these items see pages 20–23 in Chapter 3; here I give just a list.

- title or subject area
- word count
- submission date and time
- regulations for presentation
  - number of copies
  - typed or handwritten

WRITING FOR PUBLICATION

When submitting a typescript to a professional journal, it is very important to keep within the suggested word count. For a 1200 word 'slot' (about two sides of print) an editor might consider your typescript of 1350 words. Should you, however, send in something which is 3000 words long, it will probably be sent back smartly. Cutting such a submission would require too much editorial time.

Conversation with staff of both *Nursing Times* and *Nursing Standard* leaves me in no doubt that the main sin of contributors is sending in submissions which are considerably longer than that required. Such journals provide printed guidelines for their contributors, and these should be adhered to closely.

     – illustrations
     – 'academic style' required or preferred
- references
- marking scheme.

I can't resist making a couple of comments on items in this check list. First of all, don't be frightened by what might appear to be an unattainable word count. This can be, for a project, somewhere in the region of 10 000 words. Typically, students are convinced they will never reach such a staggering total. In fact, they more often have difficulty cutting out material in order not to exceed the word count.

My second comment concerns the title of your project. This might be given to you by your college, with no room for negotiation. Often, though, an assessment's topic will be given in general terms, something like: 'The client or patient with arthritis'. (I shall use this a little later to provide examples of more specific project titles.) It is then up to the student to devise her own title based on this. My plea is for a title which *tells the reader what the project is actually about*. Please try and avoid 'cute', semi-humorous titles which leave the reader in some doubt as to the subject matter of the study before him.

Establishing the boundaries

Where your college provides broad subject areas for project work, rather than specific titles, one of your first tasks should be to set yourself the boundaries, the restrictions, for your chosen project. Neglecting to do this will leave you with a very wide area of study. Just as a researcher narrows down her initial research problems so as to formulate one that is amenable to the research process, so you should tighten further and further the broad subject you've been given into a title which clearly states what is to be included in your project, and implies what is to be left out. This title then serves as a representation of the boundaries of your study.

Earlier, I gave you an example of a very broad subject: the client or patient with arthritis. As a project title this seems to me far too vague – you would need a pretty long book to cover it – and neither does it suggest the professional slant from which it is viewed (whether nurse, physiotherapist, or occupational therapist, for example). Below, therefore, I've given suggested titles which are far narrower in scope, also adding the health profession for which I feel each title is suitable.

- Safe and effective drug therapy for the elderly patient with rheumatoid arthritis. (*Medicine*)
- Drug interactions in the elderly patient with arthritis. (*Pharmacology*)
- Maintaining independence in the home for the elderly client with rheumatoid arthritis. (*Occupational therapy*)

ACTIVITY

Here are three more general health-related topics. With the help of your colleagues draw up three tightly defined titles, applicable to your own health care course, for each topic.

- Poverty and ill health.
- Changes in the NHS since 1979.
- The physically disabled client.

- Constructing a home exercise programme for a teenager with ankylosing spondylitis. (*Physiotherapy*)
- Preoperative preparation and postoperative care of an elderly patient undergoing hip replacement. (*Nursing, adult branch*)
- Depression in the elderly client with arthritis – the role of the community psychiatric nurse. (*Nursing, mental health branch*)
- Problems in dental care for the patient with an arthritic jaw. (*Dentistry*)

Reading these project titles, including those which apply to other health care professions than your own, you'll see how much more restricted they are in scope than the preliminary general subject. Taking the title that applies to your own course, you might try and tighten it even further. (For example, a student physiotherapist might restrict his project to respiratory exercises only for the teenager with arthritis of the spine.)

Remember: without tightening up your subject you risk landing yourself with a greatly increased workload, as well as producing a project which lacks structure and depth of discussion.

Planning your project

The title you devise – or which you've been given by your college – provides you with the starting point for a well-constructed project. Planning your project so that it meets the requirements of your title (without trespassing into adjacent topics) is an essential step. When discussing the writing of essays earlier, I warned about the dangers of 'free flow' writing, of putting down everything you know about a given subject. The same danger exists in project writing, but on a greatly increased scale.

By drawing up a plan first, your search through the literature is confined, allowing you to concentrate on some items while leaving others alone. You should, however, allow your literature search to guide your planning to some extent, so that you feel able to adjust your initial plan (just as a literature search helps the researcher to adjust his research questions or his chosen research tools). The process is, as you can understand, circular: you begin with a plan which guides your search through the literature, which in turn leads you back to your original plan in order to make adjustments to it. But a search without a plan is aimless, and therefore harder work and less exciting.

I'm going to draw up a plan for your consideration, based on the student physiotherapy project title given earlier. Even if your own chosen health care course is other than physiotherapy, try and follow my suggested plan in order to see how :

- it is restricted to the comparatively tight project title repeated below (in contrast to the original broad topic), and
- it nevertheless touches on broader, related aspects in order to set the scene for the project subject.

This is a difficult balancing act to follow. First you devise a satisfactorily confined title for your project. Then you decide how much background information you can safely provide without breaking out of your self-imposed boundaries. Finally, you home in on the meat of your project, the discussion of your chosen subject itself. Here, then, is the physiotherapy students' proposed title:

■ *Constructing a home exercise programme for a teenager with ankylosing spondylitis.*

Notice how the title, derived from the initial broad topic area, restricts me to a particular age-group of client and to one form of arthritis. Ankylosing spondylitis (AS) is a type of arthritis that causes pain and stiffness in the spine, typically affecting young men. I feel my project needs to include some reference to the *pathophysiology* of AS, and to forms of treatment other than exercises, but it is the latter that will form the major part of my study. (Look up the word 'pathophysiology' if you're not sure what it means.)

Here, then, is my project plan, together with a few comments:

- **Introduction:** brief description of the scope of the project, and how it links the disease (AS) with physiotherapy.
- **Pathophysiology and prognosis:** using diagrams of the normal spine and one affected by AS, a description of the disease process within the spine, other affected organs of the body, and the likely prognosis of the disease.
- **Literature review:** an overview of articles, research studies and books dealing with AS, especially those of particular relevance to physiotherapy. Point out those aspects of AS that seem most often covered by the literature, and any apparent gaps. Demonstrate how the literature has influenced the planning and content of this project.
- **Place of antiinflammatory drugs in the treatment of AS:** brief overview of actions of such drugs, their effects and common side effects, and forms in which they are delivered (orally or per rectum, for example).
- **Restrictions on AS sufferer's lifestyle:** including limiting movement of limbs and chest, chronic pain, tiredness. Effect on education, work, sexual activity, driving, self-esteem, body image.
- **Role of hospital physiotherapy department in developing exercises:** including use of hydrotherapy, limb and spine exercises, breathing exercises.
- **Role of physiotherapist in preparing AS client for discharge from direct care of physiotherapy department:** constructing an exercise programme that is individualized, practical, and likely to be followed by the client when at home. Advice about posture when standing and sitting, type of chairs in the home and school, type of bed and mattress. Use of exercise audio and video tapes.
- **Role of the National Ankylosing Spondylitis Society:** in providing encouragement, information, social contact, and funds for research.
- **Role of AS clubs:** including those run by physiotherapy departments at the client's local hospital, their role in providing encouragement and social contact.
- **Role of other health professionals:** a brief overview of the role of the client's own doctor, and perhaps a district nurse or school nurse.
- **Conclusion:** brief review of the ground covered in the project, perhaps including recommendations arising from the literature and the student's own clinical experience.
- **References**
- **Bibliography and/or recommended reading**

> **ACTIVITY**
>
> With your colleagues you should discuss this plan, noting its good points and those aspects of it with which you disagree. For example, you may feel the section on lifestyle limitation is in the wrong place. Also, is there any need for sections on drug therapy, or the role of other health professionals? You should be able to see connections between the sections on the national society and local AS clubs, and the principal subject – devising an exercise programme. Forging such links, as well as those between successive sections within the project, serves to create an internal logic and a smooth flow of ideas.
>
> Now try and create another project plan, using titles I gave earlier which relate to your health care course. If you're a student physiotherapist, don't sit back assuming I've already done yours for you! You should have been able to provide detailed criticisms of my above attempt at a plan (written as it was by a non-physiotherapist). Try replacing my teenager with AS by an elderly widower with an arthritic hip who faces a long wait for his hip replacement.

Storing and retrieving information

Figure 7.1 (p. 66) showed how one reference to the literature can lead you to another, which in turn can lead you to a third, and so on. The diagram also suggests, I think, how the information you accrue can build up into a very considerable collection. You then have a problem: how to store this information in a manner which is in itself logical, and which will aid your retrieval of it whenever you want.

There is little point in gathering lots of information pertaining to your project, if you can't later lay your hands on that particular piece of it that you need right now. Probably most of us have found ourselves hunting through our record cards, muttering, 'I *know* I've got something somewhere on . . .'

This happened to me in the preparation of a discussion paper on disability, for I knew perfectly well that I'd stored information about the percentage of disabled people in the UK population. My information at that time was stored on about 350 record cards. I looked under 'Numbers' and 'Percentage' and 'Ratio' but found nothing. It was only later, thumbing through various cards, that I accidentally found the information I'd been seeking, under 'Disabled – how many?'

I had stored this important information under a heading that was, frankly, illogical. Little wonder I couldn't lay my hands on it later.

The manner in which you store your information should ideally be decided before you begin your literature search. When storing information, you should ask yourself the question: Will I know where to look for this later? If your entire collection of information comes to no more than, say, 25 record cards, you don't have much of a problem. If, however, your project takes in many items of literature, or if it leads you to develop a particular interest in a certain subject so that you go on to collect still more material, you will need a system of information storage which is logical and helpful.

In the rest of this section I shall describe my experiences in assembling information on:

- record cards, and
- an electronic database

sharing with you both my occasional bright idea and my disasters. It is a good idea, incidentally, to compare your own system with those of your colleagues, so that each can learn from the others' mistakes.

The format I use to store information on my electronic database is the same as with my earlier record cards. There are advantages and disadvantages to both systems, and these I'll share with you later. I must confess, though, that although I am

> Store your gathered information in a manner that aids its retrieval.

enthusiastic about my computerized database, I still maintain my heavy metal box of record cards – just in case.

Record cards

Record cards, which I've mentioned in an earlier chapter, come in different sizes and colours. They are comparatively cheap and, if used intelligently, are both efficient and reasonably flexible. The key to their proper use lies, as I'll describe a little later, in the headings (the 'key words') you choose, and your use of cross-referencing.

Record cards are widely available in these sizes:

- 127 x 76 mm (5 in x 3 in)
- 152 x 101 mm (6 in x 4 in)
- 203 x 127 mm (8 in x 5 in).

Plastic storage boxes and alphabetical card dividers can be bought in each size – the bigger the size, the higher the cost. The card size I prefer is '6 by 4', big enough to contain plenty of information, and small enough to pack into a bag or briefcase for conveyance to a library or classroom.

My initial management of my record cards was not a success, because I failed to think my chosen method of information storage through. Each card was headed by the author's name and date of publication, followed by the full reference to that particular item of the literature. The rest of the card contained very brief notes on the contents of the article or book. Cards were arranged alphabetically by author.

You'll probably see the drawback immediately, more quickly than I did. Although each card contained a full reference – useful when drawing up a bibliography – retrieval of information was a huge problem. Take a card headed 'OLIVER 1988': did this contain information about definitions of disability, or were they to be found on the card headed 'FINKELSTEIN 1991'? In hunting up information I knew I had on the role of television in portraying disability issues, should I look under 'HAHN 1987' or 'RADAR 1990'? (I'll explain a little later why I use capital letters for the heading of each card.)

My only clue to the contents of each card might lie in the title of the literature. My memory served me sufficiently well to connect a particular card with a certain piece of information until my bundle of cards exceeded approximately 50. Then I was lost.

I had no choice but to devise another system, and this was one that grouped record cards under two main headings:

- one batch of cards by author and date of publication
- one batch of cards by subject matter.

I used white cards for both batches but you could, for example, keep your notes on subject matter on white cards, and your collection of references on a different coloured card. Subject matter tended to produce the larger collection of cards, because topics like POVERTY, BENEFITS, or ACCESS ran into two or more cards.

Figure 8.1 shows two cards from my collection of disability information; the top card contains the full reference to one item of the literature, with the lower card showing information in note form under the heading ACCESS, DISABLED.

The following features of this storage system should be noted:

The *author card* shows not only a full reference but also those subjects to which the author refers. Where I use capital letters, these represent the headings on subject cards, as in ACCESS, DISABLED.

Notes under *subject headings* are very brief, and are numbered. Entries in capital letters (e.g. FEWSTER 1990) tell me that the full reference is available on its own card. The asterisk (*) next to FEWSTER 1990 shows that I have a copy of this article in my files (which saves me hunting through a library for it.)

In the third entry on the ACCESS, DISABLED card, there is a cross-reference to

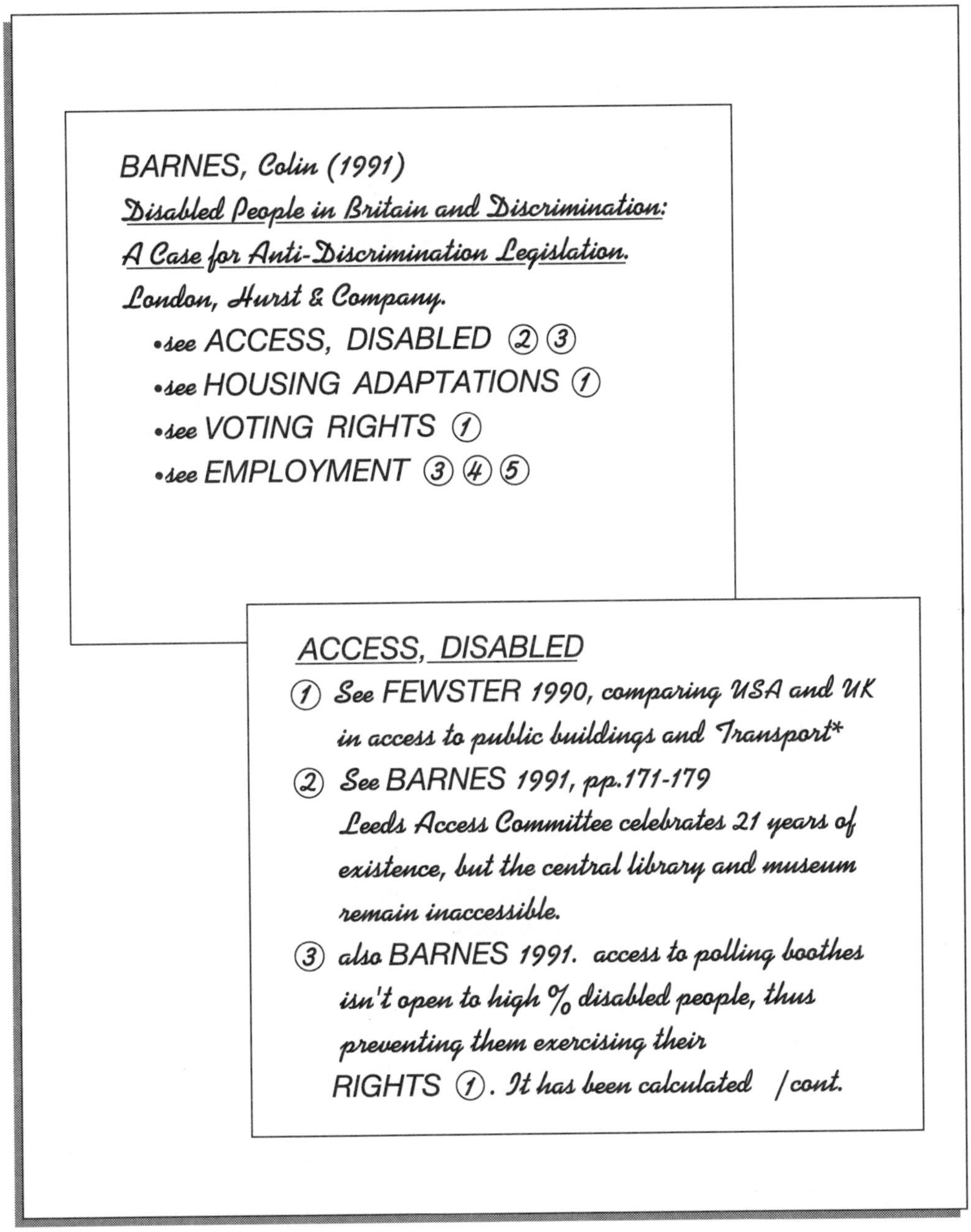

BARNES, *Colin (1991)*
Disabled People in Britain and Discrimination:
A Case for Anti-Discrimination Legislation.
London, Hurst & Company.
• *see* ACCESS, DISABLED ② ③
• *see* HOUSING ADAPTATIONS ①
• *see* VOTING RIGHTS ①
• *see* EMPLOYMENT ③ ④ ⑤

ACCESS, DISABLED
① *See FEWSTER 1990, comparing USA and UK*
*in access to public buildings and Transport**
② *See BARNES 1991, pp.171-179*
Leeds Access Committee celebrates 21 years of
existence, but the central library and museum
remain inaccessible.
③ *also BARNES 1991. access to polling boothes*
isn't open to high % disabled people, thus
preventing them exercising their
RIGHTS ①. *It has been calculated   /cont.*

Figure 8.1
Storing information on record cards
a) by author and b) by subject.
(Note the use of cross-references.)
Question – What method of
referencing is used in the top card?

VOTING RIGHTS (denoted by my use of capital letters), so that I can seek out this card for additional information. Cross-referencing is as full and as useful as you make it. Basically, the more cross-references you include, the more accessible your information is.

It is important, as I showed earlier, how you choose the key words that head each subject card. Suppose I want to gather information about disability welfare benefits. How could I store details of each of the following benefits in such a way that they could be easily found again?

> Choose 'Key
> words' with
> care in your
> information
> system.

- Mobility Allowance
- Disability Living Allowance
- Social Fund
- Attendance Allowance
- Invalidity Benefit
- Statutory Sick Pay.

Read the following notes as they might appear on a subject card. I've made them up simply to demonstrate the importance of cross-referencing. Some of the words in this passage might be regarded as useful key words, forming entries of their own on separate cards. They are important cross-references to sources of further information and so, in my system, would be written in capital letters.

■ DAILY EXPERIENCE OF DISABILITY

Frustration caused by limited access for people in wheelchairs to banks, post offices, shops, and other public buildings. Also due to insensitive attitudes of shop assistants, other shoppers, and unskilled helpers.

Particular problems for blind people are cluttered pavements (advertising boards) and road mending schemes, which need to be communicated to organizations of the blind for notification to members.

Lack of socialization arises from inability to gain access to workplace, pubs, cinemas, etc. Greater incidence of poverty among disabled also leads to isolation.

Words like ACCESS, ATTITUDES and SOCIALIZATION might serve as cross-references to other cards. Similarly, those cards would refer back to this entry. The point of cross-referencing is to guide you, like compass bearings with a map, through your stored information.

If I stored information on cards headed by the actual name of each benefit (as they appear above), I would have to remember their names in order to look them up. The word 'allowance' is common to some of them – so perhaps I could head cards with ALLOWANCE, MOBILITY and ALLOWANCE, ATTENDANCE, but that still omits other benefits.

Here are two methods that would help me search out the information in my record cards. One is to have a card headed BENEFITS listing all disability benefits by the names which head their appropriate cards. This card therefore acts as an index. First I look at the card headed Benefits (and stored in my card file under that name), in order to remind myself of the name of individual welfare benefits. From there I'm directed to the correct card for my present essay, stored under its own heading: e.g. Invalidity Benefit or Attendance Allowance.

A second method is to begin the heading of *each* card with the word BENEFIT. Thus my cards are headed:

● BENEFIT – MOBILITY ALLOWANCE
● BENEFIT – INVALIDITY BENEFIT
● BENEFIT – SOCIAL FUND

and so on.

With both of these methods, I don't need to carry around in my head the names of every disability benefit contained in my information store.

The key words you choose and your method of cross-referencing will probably make or break your card storage system.

Electronic database

Cross-referencing can be carried out in a computerized database by using its 'search' facility, as I'll show later, but the words that you use when storing information remain important to the ease with which you can later retrieve it.

When my own disability information store reached about 500 cards (350 by subject matter, 150 by author) I began to feel the need for a system that was both quicker and

---

WRITING TECHNOLOGY

When using a word processor, *always* keep a backup disk. Disks that are in constant use can be damaged, lost, stolen or erased by accident. When writing an assessment using a word processor, save what is on the screen on your disk, and its backup, at frequent intervals. A power cut is a rare event, but it almost inevitably happens when you've just finished six pages of text without bothering to store it.

---

more portable. I had already moved from a small plastic card box, which contains only about 300 cards, to a long metal box. Clearly, I needed a computer which could run a database (and one which I could readily understand and use) but, again, a keyboard and screen wouldn't fit into my briefcase.

Eventually, I chose a Psion Series 3 'palmtop' computer, both for its size and price, and for its memory capability. Casio and Sharp, among others, make cheaper versions with smaller screens and less memory; Psion themselves produce versions of their Series 3 with more memory (and at a higher price). Interestingly, the Psion is both British designed and made in Britain.

I store my disability data using the same broad divisions as with my record cards – by author and by subject. For safety, I store each set of data on a solid state disk (which isn't really a disk) and keep a backup disk as well.

Nevertheless, there are disadvantages to using an electronic database. First, it is possible to wipe out all your information by just a few key strokes. The Psion has a built-in check after you've pressed the 'Delete' key, asking you to confirm that 'delete' is what you really want to do. But once you've pressed Y (for 'Yes') your file is deleted (which is why I keep a backup disk).

Information can be lost on some small palmtops if the batteries run out, although the Psion has a backup battery which will last at least until you've changed the main batteries. It also incorporates a visual and audible warning when either battery system runs low.

Finally, someone is more likely to steal a palmtop computer worth about £200 than a plastic box containing record cards.

The principal advantage of using the Psion, or some similar machine, is its 'word search' facility. To describe this, I'm going to use another example from my disability information store.

Suppose I want to look up the information I've got on 'attacks on disabled people'. Looking at my record cards first, I find nothing under ATTACKS or DISABLED, so I turn to the palmtop and ask it to search for the word 'attack'. (I can instruct it not to bother about upper or lower case letters.) Each time the word 'attack' occurs in my electronic data – both in a document heading and its main text – that particular document is shown on the screen. Here are two examples:

1. *Attack*s on disabled by skinhead youths – a 55-year-old man died in Germany after being beaten up . . .
2. Disabled people are three times likelier to be *attack*ed in their own homes . . .

Note how only the word 'attack' is highlighted, even when it is part of a longer word like 'attacks' and 'attacked'.

Having read these two electronic documents, I remembered my record cards stored this same information under the key word GERMANY. Of course, I should have included a cross-reference card with the heading ATTACK.

For another project, I could ask the palmtop to search for words such as 'poverty', 'access', 'public transport', 'nursing care' and so on. However, there are two points worth making about this procedure.

First, my computer will only find what I've already entered. If I haven't previously put in information about nursing care of disabled people, the computer won't be able to find it.

Second, the computer will search only for the *exact word* I enter. If I misspell this word, the search facility won't realize that. It will find only the entries that are similarly misspelled.

Neither will the computer look for words that have similar meaning. If I type in 'poor', that's what the computer will search out. It won't look for 'poverty', or 'low income' or 'deprived'. It will also turn up uses of the word 'poor' that I didn't mean. To illustrate this, here are excerpts from my Psion when I asked it to search for 'poor':

1. . . . **poor** advice services available
2. . . . **poor** design of buildings
3. . . . **poor**ly adapted buildings
4. Built environment excludes disabled through **poor** access . . .

Four entries, yet not one of them relates to the meaning of 'poor' I was wanting – financially deprived. My computer can't work out what I want or mean to say. It simply carries out the instructions I give it. Neither, in this event, is it any good shouting at my computer . . .

One further disadvantage of storing documents electronically is that the computer is unable to show all the relevant documents at the same time. With record cards, you can get half a dozen spread over your desk. You can sort them into different orders and groups, your eye roving over them all at the same time. The palmtop computer cannot do this so it is much more difficult to 'shuffle the pack' (Fig. 2.5).

For speed and flexibility, as well as being a convenient small size, the palmtop has proved essential to my current disability writing. Nevertheless, it is relatively expensive and, as with all such machines, you have to spend time learning how to work it. (Mastering the Psion proved to be very easy. as its manual is exceptionally clearly written.) Without wishing to sound patronizing, record cards may well be sufficient for students on a health care course. Remember, though, those vital ingredients: logical key words and full cross-referencing. If you can, learn from my own silly mistakes, which I described earlier.

In Chapter 9, I discuss problems associated with presenting your project to your class or to another group of students.

REFERENCE
Bell J 1987 Doing your research project: a guide for first-time researchers in education and social science. Open University Press, Milton Keynes

Notes

N o t e s

9

Oral presentation of your project

Key topics

■ Interaction with a group of students
■ Practising project presentation
■ Use of overhead projectors and whiteboards

Colleges sometimes require students to present projects to their classmates. This can be an ordeal for the presenter, even where the presentation is not formally assessed. Usually, colleagues will listen positively and sympathetically, knowing all too well that it will soon be their turn to face the class. You may also like to bear in mind that facing a group of students, however large or small, is a nerve-racking experience for the new teacher or student teacher. You may find useful an article I wrote some time ago, describing my experiences as a tutor student (Goodall 1985). Perhaps you will be able to empathize with some of the feelings I described there – and therefore with the teacher who faces your class for the first time.

This chapter will also be of value for those asked to present a seminar on a given topic to a group of students.

Some colleges ask their students to undertake an oral assessment, known as a *viva voce* examination. (This term – sometimes shortened to 'viva' – comes from the Latin, 'with the living voice'; though after experiencing it you may come out feeling more dead than alive.) Some of the material contained in this chapter may be useful in your preparation for a viva voce, but it is most important for you to obtain, from your college regulations, a detailed description of the assessment's overall aims. It might be, for example, an examination of all that you've learned about human physiology or psychology. It might, however, be restricted to questioning about a written project you've submitted. Some colleges require a viva voce only where students have obtained a borderline grade in a piece of written work. The viva is then carried out to help the examiners form a definite final grade. Whatever the reason your college has for inviting you to a viva (as they so nicely express it), find out what it is first.

Problems of verbal presentation

However brief your presentation, however small your student group, it is important to try and form some sort of relationship with the people sitting in front of you. It is as well to try and avoid putting yourself forward as the expert on your subject, since this may serve to antagonize your class. Besides, you can all too easily be deflated by just one well-aimed question from your group. (Teachers might also bear this in mind.)

Your presentation should create the opportunities for questions from the group; you should make it clear at the outset whether you welcome questions throughout your presentation, or whether you'd rather they be saved till the end. If you are asked something you don't understand – or whose answer you don't at the moment know – say so. Students have a greater respect for honesty than for bluff.

Make sure your group knows the subject of your presentation from the very beginning. Don't leave them to guess. You could perhaps say how long you think your talk might last – always a sound way of reducing any signs of boredom as time proceeds.

Don't overdo humour as a means of forming a friendly relationship with your group. The occasional witty remark will help lift the atmosphere and maintain attention, but to persist in telling jokes can prove to be both tedious and fruitless. Make sure you don't upset members of your audience with insensitive humour. Be especially careful when referring to aspects of race, sex and sexuality, disability and religion. For example, if a class member fails to hear something you've said, it is unwise to ask, even with a smile, 'Are you deaf?' It could turn out that he *is*.

Practice makes perfect

It might be that you are unused to addressing a group. Anticipation is often worse than the event itself (your fright gradually draining away as you get into your stride). If you can practise your oral presentation before the actual event, you may well reduce some of that anticipatory fear.

Find out which classroom you'll be using – and think about how you'd like the chairs and desks arranged. (It's *your* presentation, so *you* decide.) Find out whether the room contains an overhead projector (OHP) and whiteboard, and whether the windows can be screened effectively.

> Avoid a delivery that is too fast and too quiet when addressing your group.

One of the main problems for students fresh to speaking before an audience is achieving an appropriate speed and volume of the voice. A common mistake for beginners, one that is increased by nervousness, is to speak too quickly. As you speak, make a conscious effort to slow down, and to make distinct pauses at the end of each sentence. Your pace may sound ridiculous to you but it won't to your audience. Volume is very difficult to achieve, especially for those with a naturally soft voice, and in large, high rooms. Even after 10 years of teaching, I still find it difficult to raise my voice sufficiently in a big room.

To help you deal with these problems take a friend, whose opinion you trust, into the same room you'll be using for your presentation. Practise giving your talk, with your friend at the back of the room. She will have detailed information from you about what she is to listen for: whether she can hear you clearly or whether she has to strain to hear (remember there will background noises, such as rustling papers, in a room full of students).

She can also listen out for personal mannerisms you might have when you speak, and of which you aren't aware. You might, for example, have an unconscious habit of ending sentences with 'OK?' or 'All right?' Once a member of your audience has spotted such idiosyncrasies, he tends to concentrate on them rather than the substance of your message. It is useful for you to be warned about such mannerisms beforehand, so that you can try to avoid them during your presentation.

Reading from a script?

When I first started teaching, my main fear was of 'drying up' in front of a class – of coming to a halt with nothing left to say. To try and get around this fear my first efforts at lesson preparation looked more like essays, so that in order to teach I simply read from my script. As I gained self-confidence, my teaching notes became more concise, containing key words, questions and references.

You may feel it is safer for you to write out your presentation word for word. There are disadvantages to this – your presentation will tend to come across as rather lifeless, because it contains no room for negotiation with your class, for sidestepping to a related subject, one that is perhaps suggested by a question from the group.

It takes considerable confidence to face an audience – even a small one – holding just a few notes in your hand. These notes then become your prompts, guiding you as you talk about your subject. You are more open to questions from your audience than where the teacher reads from a script. Related topics also emerge more easily.

If you hope to use a prompt card in your presentation, write out your notes as you would plan an essay, with headings and subheadings. I tend to use different coloured ink for noting questions, and quotations from or references to the literature. You should bear in mind that no notes, however full, can take the place of knowledge. *Know* your topic thoroughly by reading and rereading your project and related literature prior to your presentation, just as a teacher should know fully the subject he plans to teach.

Using the overhead projector (OHP)

There are several advantages to using an overhead projector (OHP) rather than a chalkboard or whiteboard. Acetates (the clear plastic sheets on which you draw and write for use with the OHP) can be prepared beforehand with as much care and thought as are available to you. As you show them, you remain facing your audience rather than turning your back, as happens when you write on a board. They can be attractively coloured (but see my notes on colour a little later) and serve to break up your verbal delivery.

One disadvantage of the OHP is the annoying humming sound it makes as its fan cools the bulb. Try not to keep an acetate showing for too long – the hotter the machine becomes, the longer the fan will run. Acetates tend to curl up if kept on the projector too long so you will need a few loose coins to hold down the edges.

A wide selection of coloured pens is available for use on acetates but do note that colours such as yellow and orange don't show up well; don't use them for printing words, although as blocks of colour they are fine. For text, use black, red, blue or purple. Green and brown show up fairly well in a darkened room, otherwise they are too pale to be effective.

Pens for OHPs use ink that is either water soluble (i.e. it can be washed off with water) or waterproof. The former are cheaper in that your acetates can be washed, dried, and reused. However, since water washes off the inks so does a sweaty hand and it is all too easy to smudge your acetate, both as you prepare them and while you're showing them. Small adjustments to waterproof ink marks on an acetate can be made by a swab soaked in spirit, or with a special eraser. As a general rule, however, waterproof acetates cannot be cleaned and reused.

Just as you tried out your voice in a classroom, try out your OHPs. Show them against a screen, then see if you can read them from the back of the room. If you can't, there is little point in showing them.

Avoid showing large blocks of text. I have known classes to be faced with an acetate consisting of a reproduced page of printed text – a complete waste of time and money because none of it could be read. It simply served to antagonize the audience. Ideally, each acetate should show one basic idea in an eye-catching way. For example, to get across the idea of barriers to communication between nurse and patient, you might draw a patient in bed and a nurse, separated by a brick wall.

Before your seminar or project presentation, check the OHP you'll be using. Check that the bulb works and that the lens is free of dust. Think about the arrangement of

> Always ensure your OHP acetates are visible from the back of the classroom.

chairs in your classroom, ensuring that everyone will be able to see your OHP. Check the window curtains or blinds for their effectiveness at blocking out the light.

Ask your friend or colleague to hear your whole presentation, noting whether your acetates appear at an appropriate place. Do they manage to make a point concisely and effectively? Could that point be better made using some other visual aid?

Using a whiteboard

Because you have to turn away from your audience to write on the board, you could consider asking a member of your audience (or a co-presenter) to act as your scribe. Another method is to prepare your whiteboard beforehand, writing concise points or helpful diagrams before your audience arrives. However you choose to use it, the whiteboard helps to break up your delivery, just as the OHP does.

Be careful about which pens you use. Whiteboards use special pens whose ink can be easily rubbed off afterwards. Your college may not thank you for using the wrong type of pen with indelible ink.

Either whiteboards or large-sized sheets of paper may be used to resource small-group work that you incorporate in your presentation. Here, each group will need its own whiteboard, paper sheet(s) and pens. If you plan to use group work, be sure you provide clear instructions about what the groups should achieve. Preferably hand each group a card giving written instructions, together with their time limit. Ensure there is sufficient space (for example, spare empty classrooms) for groups to work in undisturbed by each other.

Handouts

Providing handouts can be useful for getting across an overview of your presentation, as well as important references. Telling your class at the beginning of your talk that handouts are available sometimes helps students decide whether or not they need to take notes. Students seem to find handouts reassuring, in that they have something tangible to take away from the class (rather like a patient getting a prescription from his GP).

However, I sometimes wonder about the value of handouts. It seems to me that, where they are provided, they tend to go straight into students' files – unread. But that is the responsibility of those students, not you.

When it's all over

After your presentation, after the applause has died away, find the time to write a few notes about what happened (just as, ideally, a teacher should after a class). You will have fresh in your mind the moments that went well and those that were a bit sticky. Why were the latter problematic? Was it that you weren't absolutely clear in your mind about your facts? Or was there an interruption in the class, or the OHP bulb blew, or a student asked a particularly difficult question?

Why did other parts of your presentation go smoothly? You should strive to be critically aware of your presentation, not just relieved that it's all over. If one particular aspect of the talk was excellent, try and understand why. We can learn as much from good events in the classroom as from bad.

Can you assess the quality of your interaction with the class? How attentively did the students appear to listen, how did they respond to your questions and to the

> **ACTIVITY**
>
> It is challenging, but worthwhile, evaluating a class that one has given, even (perhaps especially) when it is a session that a teacher has given many times before. Now that you have survived your presentation, and probably found it not as bad as you anticipated, work out how you might evaluate your session by discovering the students' reactions to it. You could perhaps devise a brief evaluation sheet that could be handed out to students after the class.

OHP, and were there some points that seemed to provoke puzzlement, or do you think you got everything across well?

What I've just described here, and what I suggest in the above activity box, is a form of *reflective practice*. I'm suggesting that it is valuable for everyone involved in health care – student or registered practitioner, bedside nurse or teacher – to reflect critically on her own daily performance. In Chapter 12, there is a brief discussion about this with regard to ward- or field-based practical work, and I include the suggestion there that you keep a learning journal or log as part of your personal and professional development. (Your health care course might *require* you to keep such a journal, though if this is not the case I would strongly urge you to consider doing so of your own accord.)

Journals or diaries relating to one's work need to be completed, preferably, immediately after the event being described, otherwise some of the important detail is forgotten. They also need to be self-critical – which, as I've pointed out several times before, does *not* exclude praise. If you can develop headings for your personal learning journal to help you focus on important events, and your reactions to them, so much the better.

Learning logs (which is my preferred term for a diary or journal) can be applied not just to ward work, or fieldwork in the community, but to essay writing and carrying out a literature search for a project, and even to writing articles for publication. There is nothing quite so salutary as forcing yourself to analyse what has gone wrong (or right) with a particular section of an article or chapter – unless it's listening to your editor telling you what you ought to have worked out for yourself.

REFERENCE
Goodall C 1985 A student tutor's evaluation of his teaching placement. Nurse Education Today 5: 95–100

Notes

10 Writing a research critique

Key points

■ The nature and process of research
■ The place of research in health care professions
■ Questions to ask of published research

There is nothing mysterious about research. Research is a process that requires clear thinking rather than any particularly advanced mental gymnastics. Research might be described as the clear definition of a problem, followed by the methodical investigation of that problem, and the promulgation of its results at conferences, in lectures, or by publication. That last point is, I believe, especially important. If a research study establishes means of improving client care, it needs to be read by those who can put it into action.

Compared with medicine, nursing has turned to research comparatively late, in an attempt to challenge and discard much of its care that was based on little but myth. The emphasis on research, both in nursing publications and in nurse education, may perhaps have served to frighten the very students and nurse practitioners it most sought to inform. Nevertheless, such a challenge was probably necessary. Health professionals, rather than delivering care 'off the peg', need to be equipped to challenge their own interventions: what am I doing to his patient and why? How can I justify the care I'm giving? How better might this be performed? To embrace research-based care is to put yourself in the uncomfortable position of constantly questioning the care you deliver.

How to carry out research is beyond the scope of this chapter. Instead, I discuss a student assessment that is a requirement of many health care courses – writing a critique of a published piece of research. For this assessment, students probably require as clear an appreciation of the *process* of research (rather than its intricate details) as if they were doing research for themselves.

Ogier (1989) provides a clear introduction to the critical reading of nursing research, while Hockey (1985) is both informative and informal. For those who have to produce their own research study, I recommend Bell (1987), and for a discussion of the research process as it applies to nursing, then both Cormack (1991) and Burnard & Morrison (1990) are excellent texts. Statistical tests are explored in detail in Hicks (1990) again with a slant towards nursing. For students who are interested in qualitative research, Cormack (1991) provides a good introduction, after which Strauss & Corbin (1990) could be tried.

Many of the Royal College of Nursing monographs provide useful examples of how research studies are laid out, and by quickly reading through two or three of these you can gain some idea of what research 'feels' like. Perhaps you will be tempted to go straight to the 'Conclusions' and 'Recommendations' sections, since there you'll find the pointers to help improve your nursing care, but it is important also to gain an idea of the basis for those recommendations. How were they arrived at by the researcher? Are they appropriate conclusions? Can they be applied to other health care settings? Only by appreciating the whole research study can these important questions be answered.

There is no assumption that each nurse, physiotherapist, or occupational therapist should engage in carrying out research in their professional roles. But it is reasonable to expect that every health professional should be research-conscious, and aware of its place in enhancing care. There should be a willingness, as well as an ability, to read research, evaluate it, and, where appropriate, apply it.

All that glitters

Several misconceptions have emerged so often during my experience of marking research critiques that I was tempted to ask whether students' education about research was sufficient for them to carry out the required assessment. Other teachers' experiences may be different, but I share mine with you here to help you avoid similar mistakes.

The first misconception is to equate 'research' with any article that appears in a professional journal. An understanding of the actual process of research would soon dispel this belief but it is one that seems to occur commonly. Thus I have read, of one of my own articles, that 'Goodall (1988) has proved that chronic pain produces a different attitude to daily life than does acute pain'. No he doesn't – he merely puts forward his view that this is the case. Goodall (1988) is purely anecdotal, though it is none the worse for that.

> A study is not a piece of research simply because it is published. There is a *process* of research that must be followed by the investigator.

The second misconception is that all research must begin with a hypothesis. Students seem to seize on this word out of all that they've learned and read about research, and deem it to be of such central importance that it must occur in all research papers. Consequently they label something as a 'hypothesis' when it isn't anything of the sort. One reason for this may be, as Hunt suggests, that in nursing there has been a bias towards quantitative research, with qualitative research regarded as being of a lower status (Hunt 1991). Much quantitative research (but not all) sets out to test a hypothesis, whereas probably all research tries to address the research *question* posed at the beginning of each study. A research question is not the same as a hypothesis.

ACTIVITY

It may be useful for you at this point to investigate the basic differences between quantitative and qualitative research, and then to discuss your findings with your colleagues. Can you give examples of each? Why do you think it may be that the latter had, until recently, a lesser reputation than the former? On what other fields of study was the early quantitative nursing research in this country based?

Secondly, try and discover what is a hypothesis, and again find examples in various research papers. In what type of research does a hypothesis occur? In what type of research would you not expect to find a hypothesis, and why?

The third misconception seems to be that all research worth its salt must contain a questionnaire. This wouldn't be such a fatal mistake to make, if composing questionnaires wasn't so fraught with peril for the inexperienced researcher. Yet I have certainly come across students who feel that, if they don't include a questionnaire, their research isn't of any value.

Now, all three misconceptions above are *anecdotal*: they've arisen out of my marking and tutorial experience, and not out of educational research. Other teachers may have different student misconceptions to report. But I can certainly say that those misconceptions I came across were firmly held.

The process of research

> It is the nature of the initial research that guides the researcher's choice of a suitable methodology.

There is a step-by-step process to conducting research, one that helps to identify a study as research-based rather than as, say, a review of the writer's beliefs. A student's critique of a piece of research that follows this process would seem to me to be soundly based. The research process is shown, in simplified form, in Figure 10.1, though for more detailed information you could try Chapter 7 in Cormack (1991).

In examining Figure 10.1, you may wonder why the research process is represented as some sort of inward-moving spiral. This shape was chosen to represent how, often, a researcher begins with a problem that is expressed rather loosely, but whose subsequent investigations serve to focus on this problem more and more tightly. When you begin your research, you feel as if you're prowling round the outer edges of a field, getting an overview of what that field contains. Then you notice certain details, and choose some for closer examination, while discarding others. Thus you move from the edges of the field towards the middle, getting closer to the tightly-defined central issue. This process was, I felt, better represented by a spiral figure rather than by one that appeared to be simply linear.

Asking questions

You would do well, initially, to seek your tutor's advice in picking an appropriate published research study on which to base your critique, so that you don't end up with one that is far too complex. In order to discuss critically your chosen piece of research (and remember that to criticize means you may praise as well as find fault)

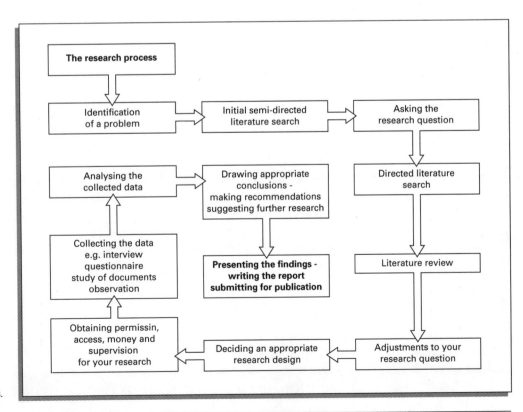

Figure 10.1
An overview of the research process.

> It is always a good idea, when reading published articles and research studies, to question the views or assertions of the author. Try and form the habit of reading *critically*.

one scheme you can follow is to ask a series of questions about it. These questions can broadly reflect the research process, as outlined above.

Here I give you some suggested questions, together with comments on each, but please don't treat them as a rigid check list through which to work. Discuss them first with colleagues in your group who are doing the same assessment as yourself. There are doubtless improvements you will be able to make to my suggestions, as well as additions.

1. Is the research title helpful?

I have earlier commented on the use and misuse of titles for studies and projects, so you will already know my views about those titles that might be described as 'cute'. To my mind, a title should tell you what the piece of work is about. It should help you to decide whether it is something you would do well to follow up, or to leave alone. Picturesque and poetic titles would be better reserved for your first novel.

2. Is this research useful to me as a professional?

As someone whose distant PhD thesis was on some nebulous aspect of musicology, I may be better qualified than many to suggest that health care research should be *applicable*. You could ask: how might this research help me to care for my patient or client? How might it help me educate patients, or improve the learning of student physiotherapists? What does it tell me about the human condition that is not just interesting, but useful?

A sociologist might, for instance, wish to carry out a study into the percentage of male student nurses who are left wing. This could, I suppose, be regarded as interesting, since it would tell us something about the political views of men who decide to enter one of the caring professions. But does it help the business of caring? Somehow, I doubt it. (You might also ponder the problem of how a researcher could go about finding the necessary data for his study. The more personal the questions asked, in interviews or questionnaires – for example, concerning a person's sexual activity or orientation – the less likely, I suppose, it is that honest answers would be forthcoming.)

By contrast, research into the sickness/absence rate among registered nurses has direct implications for the management of hospital and community services. Do new staff nurses have more or less time off sick than ward managers or district nurses? Have the widespread health service changes brought about an increase in sickness levels among nurses and other health professions? What are the reasons behind much sickness? These are questions well worth investigating, I would suggest. They are of practical value.

3. What research question is asked by this study?

> Don't expect to find a *hypothesis* in every piece of research. In what type of research would you look for an hypothesis?

The researcher will have started off with a research problem, something that has nagged her in her professional practice, and from this her research question will have been formulated. An example of such a question might be, 'Has the sickness/absence rate among trained nurses risen significantly over the past 3 years?' Only in certain types of research, remember, will this question be reworked into a hypothesis, so here is a supplementary question to ask of your chosen piece of research: Is there a hypothesis that this study sets out to test?

4. Does the research replicate an earlier study?

I initially believed that research had to be original to be of any worth, and certainly original work pushes back the boundaries of knowledge. But equally valuable is the research that replicates (repeats) a study carried out earlier. For example, you might come across research carried out in 1983 in a Newcastle teaching hospital on levels of sickness among newly appointed occupational therapists. Now, how applicable is that study to your own situation in rural Kent? And do its findings hold true for today? Would it apply to newly appointed physiotherapists or house officers? To find out, the study would need replication, perhaps involving three or four district hospitals in the south of England (rather than one northern teaching hospital).

5. Does the literature review influence the design or direction of the study?

Judge the literature review not by the abundance of references found there but by the level of discussion. The researcher will have gathered examples of earlier research, and will have demonstrated areas of her subject where research abounds and other areas where there is a deficit. Has any preceding research led the writer to adjust her research focus or methodology? Has the research question itself been adjusted because of previous research discussed in the literature review? Was there a related study which caused the researcher to include, say, interviews as well as questionnaires? In brief, what is the *link* between the literature review and the research study you are critiquing?

6. What broad type of research is my chosen study?

For example, is it quantitative or qualitative? Does it use an experimental approach – altering one 'variable' (e.g. the type of physiotherapy applied to patients with rheumatoid arthritis in the hands) in order to see if another variable changes (e.g. the amount of pain experienced by the patient or the level of manual dexterity achieved).

Perhaps your study could be described as 'action research' whereby the researcher, a nurse in a busy accident service, carries out an investigation in his own professional sphere, in order to facilitate changes. (Incidentally, as a student therapist or nurse, you might find the concept of action research a particularly attractive and useful one. The researcher is perceived not as an expert imposing his findings but as a participant, working with and for members of his team. It is an attempt to cross the gap that is often perceived to exist between the theory of research and its practical application.)

7. What research tools are used?

This is perhaps the most complex area of study for someone appraising a piece of research. Consideration of the various research tools – such as interviews, questionnaires, examination of documents, observation – is beyond the scope of this chapter. You may at first feel that it is not for you to approve or question the design of a published study, but within the limitations of your familiarity with research methods it is nevertheless possible to make intelligent comments. You will be able to identify which tools are used, and some of the drawbacks and advantages associated with their use.

For example, in making observations on a ward, it is possible for the researcher to affect the results of her investigations. Supposing a researcher tells the ward staff she is observing the quality of the patients' reports during shift handovers, those nurses – with the researcher nearby clutching her clipboard – will make every effort to provide high quality communication. In other words, the investigator has herself influenced the very data she is collecting.

If a questionnaire has been employed, you can discover whether it has been tested on a small group of respondents first in a pilot study, in order to help iron out any ambiguities in the questions asked. You can discover what sort of replies are elicited from the questions – are respondents asked to tick boxes, to put items in order of priority, or to write brief replies of their own? Is there space for respondents to enlarge on their answers? (In completing questionnaires myself, I sometimes feel my answers should begin, 'Yes, but . . . ', because none of the provided replies seems

> Are questionnaires formulated in such a way that they invite answers that are both honest and accurate?

adequate.) Are respondents assured of their anonymity being preserved? If the researcher is a member of management, are such assurances likely to be believed by junior staff? (This is not to suggest that assurances of anonymity, given by a manager-researcher, are worthless. The problem lies with how those assurances are *perceived* by the study's respondents.)

Suppose, for example, I am investigating stress among student nurses, I may include in my questionnaire the item: 'Have you ever taken time off sick when you were not genuinely ill?' The problem with this naive question is whether it is likely to gain an honest answer, especially when my respondents know me as a teacher in their college, and thus a member (in their eyes) of the hierarchy. Incidentally, you may wonder what is meant by that word 'genuinely' in this context. Aren't stress and anxiety about a student's ward placement 'genuine' manifestations of ill health?

As a researcher, you have to rely on your respondents – both to questionnaires and to interviews – replying honestly. They may have many reasons for not providing you with an honest answer – they don't like you, they don't like researchers, they want to protect themselves and their future prospects of employment, or they are anxious to 'help' you by giving you the answer they think you want. You also have to construct your questions in such a way that they are absolutely clear, hence the importance of a pilot study in which a questionnaire is tested. A researcher once commented to me, 'I only find out exactly what I've asked when the replies come back' – a very honest statement to make.

8. Do the results and their associated recommendations (if any) derive appropriately from the data collected?

One danger in carrying out research, is believing you know beforehand what are the solutions to the problem you're investigating. We'll come across an example of this in the activity box that ends this chapter. Where a researcher sets out to investigate a problem, and where he is sure beforehand what his research will show and what the appropriate solutions are, the possibility exists that the researcher will swing his results in such a way that they back up his beliefs.

Suppose a college manager believes her teachers have grossly unequal workloads, and she wishes to show that this is so. She examines class timetables over the previous 3 months for information about the teaching hours of her staff. She finds that, in week 7, Miss Jones taught for 5 hours, whereas Mr Edwards taught for 8 hours. From this and similar data the manager claims that teacher workloads are indeed unequal. She has proved her beliefs to be correct – but is this actually the case? No – the documentation studied tells the researcher nothing about time spent, for example, in lesson preparation, marking, holding tutorials, visiting wards, reading in the college library or counselling anxious students, and so on. The manager's claims outstrip the data collected. The only conclusion that can be drawn from data on teaching hours is a comparison of timetabled teaching. It would not even be safe to assume that more timetabled teaching hours equated with more teacher time spent in lesson preparation. A lesson lasting 2 hours may be one that has already been well prepared. In this imaginary situation, because the college manager set out to collect data that would prove her beliefs to be correct, she (purposely?) omitted to study data that might challenge them.

Research that examines aspects of care will likely include recommendations for practice. You should ask whether all of these derive appropriately from the data which is presented to the reader, and also whether they could apply to other situations. Research into the assessment of pain experienced by patients following surgery will produce results that might not safely apply to patients living at home with chronic pain, or to the pain experienced by young children.

You should ascertain how large a sample the researcher uses in his study, and whether this allows him safely to make recommendations. For example, if my research included a questionnaire sent to five ward managers, of whom three replied, I could not justifiably make any useful recommendations to the whole nursing staff, or even to all the 56 ward managers in my large hospital.

When I read a piece of research by skipping the difficult parts and going straight to the findings and recommendations, I am backing away from being able to judge the validity of those recommendations. Certainly, no practitioner should put into practice any research findings without ensuring that they are appropriately made from the data collected.

Such judgements are difficult to make without the necessary educational background of research appreciation. However, by attending local research interest groups, for example, you can listen to discussions about various studies and their appropriateness for action, as well as meeting others, like yourself, who find research both difficult and fascinating. As you gain familiarity with the terminology, you also gain in appreciating the enormous benefits of research to health care. You may also gain the confidence to suggest, and carry out, your own research.

> Results and recommendations are important features of the research process, but the reader must ascertain their validity before applying them to her own clinical area.

9. Are there suggestions for further research?

No piece of research is the end of the story. There is always something new to be investigated. It is a mark of the investigator's research awareness – not of his humility – to suggest gaps in his own study, and associated areas that could be studied by those following on. 'I have investigated X', he may write, 'but although the possibility of Y occurred to me, there was neither the time nor the resources to cover further research. Therefore Y remains to be studied.'

10. How clearly is the study expressed?

It is useful to gain a general impression about your chosen study's reader-friendliness. You may comment about the clarity of its writing, not just the use of specialist vocabulary that the writer deems necessary to the expression of exact ideas, but also those occurrences (if any) where the language used seems to serve merely to baffle. You may also comment on how much any tables or figures contribute to the communication of facts. Are the figures well drawn and adequately captioned? Do they require detailed reading of the main text before their relevance can be grasped? You may also ask: What purpose does this particular figure serve? Does it explain the text, and add to it usefully, or does it appear without any apparent relevance to the text? I have explored clarity and accuracy of expression in reseach, as well as the nature of research, in the journal *Nurse Researcher* (Goodall 1994). In that paper, I argued for clear communication of research findings as a vital part of the research process itself.

All of the above 10 questions could be answered without detailed knowledge of the deeper intricacies of research. Yet I would suggest that they could be answered sufficiently well to provide an informed and intelligent evaluation of your chosen research study. By answering these questions, as well as others that occur to you, you can demonstrate that you have grasped the essentials of the process of research, and have the ability to make some judgement about the relevance of your chosen study to your sphere of professional practice.

The remainder of this chapter is devoted to an activity box, one that is a little longer than usual. It consists of a research report, specially written for this chapter, which contains certain recommendations that, initially, might appear both obvious and correct. After you've read the report, however, you may feel inclined to disagree with the conclusions of the imagined researcher. There are several questionable statements in the text, and at these points I've inserted a number in square brackets, like this [4]. At the end, next to the appropriate number, I've made brief comments; but I'm going to leave the 'meat' of the criticisms to you.

The report is very much shorter than would normally be the case following a period of research.

A STITCH IN TIME [1]

Introduction

Managers of the Anytown NHS Hospital Trust have become increasingly concerned about the rising incidence of needle-stick injury among hospital staff, especially nurses. Such injuries have obvious implications for staff ill health, with loss of time from work, and also for financial claims on the Trust. Therefore, the Chief Executive requested me to undertake research into the actual incidence of injury, in order to assess the size of the problem and to suggest which groups of staff require additional education and safety training [2].

Methodology [3]

The method chosen for investigating the problem was an examination of Accidents To Staff Forms (ATSF) over the past year in all wards and departments of the hospital. Forms from the community were not included. Figures were collected of needle-stick injuries, and were catalogued according to the type and grade of staff involved.[4]

Findings

Over the year, 46 ATSFs were discovered that related to hospital staff needle-stick injury. On only 30 forms was it clearly stated at which stage of the injection procedure the injury occurred, [5] that is, either pre-injection or post-injection.

The profession and grade of staff to which injury occurred is shown in Table 1. Three needle-stick injuries happened to registered nurses at staff nurse level; only one house officer suffered an injury (and no other grade of doctor); while 42 injuries involved student nurses. None of the ATSFs stated the students' year of training.

Table 1. Number of needle-stick injuries and grade of staff involved

Staff grade	Number/injuries
House officer	1
Registrar	0
Ward Manager	0
Staff nurse	3
Student nurse	42
Total injuries	46

Conclusions and recommendations

It is possible to draw only one conclusion from these results, and that is that training and education in personal safety while drawing up and giving injections is totally inadequate among student nurses. [6] This report, following discussion by the Trust Executive Management Committee, will be forwarded to the Director of Nursing Studies for consideration and immediate action. [7]

As regards trained nurses, it seems sufficient to circulate a memo drawing their attention to the Trust's policy regarding the giving of injections, and emphasizing the importance of following that policy to the letter.

Comments

[1]. How helpful do you find this title?

[2]. Is it appropriate to state, at this stage of the investigation, what the answer to the problem is?

[3]. There is no literature review in this study. Does this matter in such a restricted research setting? What might a search of the literature have revealed, and how might it have influenced the research?

[4]. One research tool has been chosen. Are there any other tools that might have revealed useful information?

[5]. Perhaps this finding should lead to its own recommendation a little later in the report.

[6]. I disagree, and for two reasons which I'll hint at by asking the following two questions:
   a. How useful do you think 'raw scores' are (as given in the report), compared with, for example, the percentages of injured staff of their clinical grade?
   b. Out of ward managers, staff nurses, and student nurses, who do you think is most likely actually to handle the syringe and needle before, during and after the injection? Would this influence the findings at all?

[7]. There is no suggestion for further research. The personnel manager, having strongly demanded additional safety training for student nurses, might have considered running a follow-up study. What might this have investigated?

The background to the report is as follows. A hospital trust chief executive is concerned at the apparently rising number of needle-stick injuries among nursing staff, and so she requests her personnel manager to carry out some research into which staff are most at risk, and what steps need to be taken to reduce the incidence of injury. (Needle-stick injuries, by the way, occur when a needle is accidentally jabbed into a nurse's or doctor's finger, either during drawing up an injection, or after it has been given and the needle and syringe are being cleared away. The latter, where the needle has been withdrawn from the patient, is the more serious because of the risk of hepatitis and HIV transmission.)

Here then, on the left hand page, is the personnel manager's brief report of his research.

REFERENCES AND RECOMMENDED READING
Bell J 1987 Doing your research project: a guide for first-time researchers in education and social sciences. Open University Press, Milton Keynes
Burnard P, Morrison P 1990 Nursing research in action: developing basic skills. Macmillan Press, London
Cormack D (ed) 1991 The research process in nursing. 2nd edn. Blackwell Scientific Publications, Oxford
Goodall C 1988 Living with pain. Nursing Times 84 (32): 62–63
Goodall C 1994 Writing and research: an introduction. Nurse Researcher 2 (1): 4–12
Hicks C 1990 Research and statistics: a practical introduction for nurses. Prentice Hall, Hemel Hempstead
Hockey L 1985 Nursing research – mistakes and misconceptions. Churchill Livingstone, Edinburgh
Hunt M 1991 Qualitative research. In: Cormack D (ed) 1991 The research process in nursing. 2nd edn. Blackwell Scientific Publications, Oxford p. 117
Ogier M 1989 Reading research. Scutari Press, London
Strauss A, Corbin J 1990 Basic of qualitative research: grounded theory procedures and techniques. Sage Publications, California

N o t e s

11 The unseen examination

Key points

■ Revising actively for examinations
■ Important words used in examination questions
■ Practising answering examination questions

Although I have usually done well for myself out of exams, I should begin by confessing that I am not their greatest fan. You must forgive me, therefore, if this chapter does not ring with loud praise for this form of student assessment. I have misgivings about their effectiveness in testing a student's knowledge and her ability to focus her thoughts on a given subject. Given the wide range of a health profession curriculum, it is impossible for one or two exam papers, sat at the end of the academic course, to address all topics. Therefore the student's knowledge of at least some important subjects will remain untested by examination.

I am especially doubtful about the 'performance' aspect of sitting exams: that on a certain date, at a certain time, in a certain place, you shall deliver yourself of high quality work for the benefit of the marker and your own career. Why? A concert pianist has to perform at a set time and place (so that he and his audience coincide) but not, surely, a student nurse or therapist. Performing to your best ability (or at least sufficiently well to gain a pass grade) at a fixed date and time takes no account of students with colds or hay fever, or any other personal problem that affects the quality of their work.

Neither can I see the point in limiting the time available for a student to compose his answer. I quite see the importance of a student nurse knowing how to work swiftly under pressure – during a cardiac arrest, for example, or admitting a patient with acute retention of urine. But to restrict him to 35 minutes when he is writing about, say, poverty and ill health, is as logical as requiring the pianist to get through a Brahms piano concerto in 35 minutes. (Note: the usual time is about 48 minutes.)

Grudgingly I concede that the prospect of exams can prove to be a useful motivator for persuading students to work hard, though whether exams are a greater prompt than, say, care studies or essays, I am unsure. Nevertheless, many colleges' assessment strategies include one or more examinations, especially towards the end of a course, and it is essential for the student to know how to prepare for them.

The marking process

Students sometimes categorize teachers according to their approach to marking, with some regarded as 'easy' markers and others as 'hard'. It follows from this that whether you pass your exams depends to some extent on the marker you get. Such a fatalistic view, however, is misplaced. Let me assure you that the system of internal and external moderation serves to iron out any great discrepancies between the standards of different markers.

Internal moderation takes the form of a second college marker reviewing the marks awarded by the first. In my college, it is the rule that the first marker must not write comments on the exam scripts themselves so that these do not influence the second marker's decision. Where the two college markers disagree about a mark, the script is passed to the external moderator – usually an experienced teacher from another college. Most usually, however, the two internal markers can discuss their scripts and arrive at a joint decision.

The external moderator will review all papers that have failed or that are borderline. He will also see a percentage of other papers in order to judge the overall standard of marking. He may, for example, ask to see papers that have received very high marks, together with some that have been awarded average marks.

The whole point of moderation is to rule out any influence – benign or malignant – of an individual marker. No single marker will make the decision to fail a script. Usually, a script that attains a fail grade will have been seen by no less than three markers.

Incidentally, I should point out that it is almost always the case that markers *want to pass students*. If a script looks doubtful, each marker will search for any possible excuse for awarding a few extra marks. No pleasure, believe me, is gained by failing students, since the markers know full well of the effects failure may have on a student's professional future, as well as his self-esteem.

Markers are provided with answer guides for each question – not so much model answers, but overviews of the main points the student is expected to include. There will also be provided a scheme which shows how marks are to be awarded – for organization of the answer, for spelling and grammar, for clinical accuracy, for inclusion of references to the literature and to the student's own practical placements.

It is important for colleges to inform their students of such marking schemes. For example, if 20% of the marks are awarded for references to the literature, the students must be aware of this.

Important instructions

You will remember that when I discussed writing essays and projects, I mentioned a number of important instructions relating to your assessment about which you must be clear before planning your work – things such as submission date and word count. There are similar instructions relating to an exam paper.

> *Before* you take your exam, be clear how many questions you must answer, and how much time you're allowed. Double check the date and time of each exam, and the hall where it is held.

Well before sitting an exam – even while you're revising for it and practising writing answers – you should know clearly how much time you are allowed for each paper. The maximum length of time for a single paper is usually 3 hours, but your exam might be 2 or $2\frac{1}{2}$. Knowing in advance how much time you have, will allow you to plan the way you allocate time within the paper for planning and writing each answer.

You should note how many questions you must attempt, and how those questions are divided (if at all) on the paper. You may, for example, be asked to attempt a total of four questions out of seven: two questions from Section A, and a further two from Section B.

You should be aware of your college's regulations relating to a student who fails to attempt the correct number of questions. Where a student hands in three answers rather than four, it might be the case that her script will not be marked, but instead will automatically be awarded a fail grade. Where such a script is marked, the student will have reduced the total possible marks she can gain from 100 to 75.

All this seems very obvious, yet many markers will tell you of students who fail to observe even the most basic exam instructions. At that feared moment when you're allowed to turn over the exam paper, and the clock starts to tick towards the finish, it is all too easy to skip the instructions at the head of the paper and go straight to the 'meat' – the questions themselves. It is in this way that fatal errors can occur. Teachers should provide their students with 'mock' papers, not only so that they can practise writing answers, but also so that they can familiarize themselves with the exam instructions for each paper they sit.

Perhaps of less immediate interest to you, but still important, your college will have drawn up regulations regarding untoward incidents in the examination hall: someone being taken ill during an exam, or a fire alarm sounding. There are also instructions to the invigilator who suspects a student of cheating. Be very careful indeed not to take into the exam room pieces of scrap paper which could be mistaken by your invigilator for memoranda. Likewise, avoid the temptation to whisper comments about the paper under your breath, either to yourself or to your friend at the next desk.

The vocabulary of exams

Each word in an examination question is important. Every question will have been debated by an examination board so that its effectiveness in testing knowledge can be judged, and any ambiguities ironed out. Questions often contain 'command' words that will tell you how to plan your answer: words such as compare, contrast, discuss, describe, list and outline. You need to be clear exactly what is meant by these commands. Sometimes colleges will issue lists of such commands with their own interpretation, and such lists will be available to students and markers. Here I comment on just a few important terms.

Compare and contrast

Here you are asked to state aspects of the given topic which are similar and those that are dissimilar. Your question might, for example, ask you to compare and contrast the state of the NHS in the 1990s with that at its inception. You could *compare* the declared aim of the NHS in both given periods to provide care which is free at the point of delivery. Then you could *contrast* the items of care which actually were free in 1948 and for which the patient now has to pay. Both command words need to be addressed by your answer if they both appear in the question. (These two words are often linked within a question.)

Describe and discuss

The Collins English Dictionary (1991) defines 'describe' as 'to give an account or representation of in words'. In other words, to describe something – a building, a picture, an aspect of care – you state its appearance, what it is that you see. In describing, for example, the postoperative care of Mrs Meredith who has had her gallbladder removed, you might include the giving of a pain killing injection:

■ *'Mrs Meredith was observed for signs of pain following her operation, and she was given 75 mg of pethidine as prescribed by the doctor. The nurse then noted the effectiveness of the injection. A vomit bowl and tissues were placed nearby.'*

To *discuss* is to explore an issue more deeply. The Collins Dictionary gives the origin of the word as coming from the Latin: to examine, to investigate, and even 'to dash to pieces'. Presumably that last could be taken to mean: picking the given subject to pieces in order to examine it in greater detail. To discuss is to do more than simply state something's appearance, as with 'describe'. This is how I might *discuss* the provision of pain relief for Mrs Meredith following her cholecystectomy:

■ *'In order to prevent Mrs Meredith experiencing postoperative pain, she was given an injection of pethidine 75 mg as prescribed by the doctor. This comparatively low dose was prescribed because Mrs Meredith weighed only 58 kilograms. The nurse observed Mrs Meredith following the injection for signs of its effectiveness. He also monitored the patient's respiration rate, because pethidine can depress a patient's breathing. A vomit bowl and some tissues were placed within Mrs Meredith's reach since pethidine can also cause nausea and vomiting. Mrs Meredith had earlier told the nurse that morphine caused her great nausea; this is why the doctor chose pethidine as her analgesic.'*

> One way in which you can *discuss* something, such as patient care, is to give the reasons for choosing that care, or to provide alternative approaches to care. To discuss is deeper than to describe.

Can you see the difference? To *describe* the patient's care means stating what happens, what an observer might see the nurse do for the patient. To *discuss* is to include reasons for the care given. My discussion of Mrs Meredith's care includes no more items of care than does my description; but instead involves a more detailed examination of what occurs. It follows, therefore, that to discuss is a lengthier process than to describe, and your examiners will bear this in mind when composing questions.

List and outline

You don't need a dictionary definition for 'list', but students certainly seem to need reassuring that when the word appears in a question, all they are required to do is – *list*! A question might incorporate the following: 'List the side effects of pethidine'. To answer this, you simply state, either in single words or very brief phrases, all the side effects you can think of. Then it needs some nerve on your part to leave your list well alone and move on to the next part of the question. To answer such a question with more details than are wanted is to waste time which would be better spent on the next question or part.

You could apply the word 'outline' to the same sort of question: 'Outline the side effects of pethidine.' Here you use one or two brief sentences for each side effect, rather than one or two words, in order to furnish some explanation. Either 'list' and 'outline' would probably appear in a short answer exam paper, or the first part of a longer question.

Using a problem-solving approach

This form of wording became popular in nursing exams as a reaction against those questions requiring student nurses to describe or discuss the treatment of a disease such as a heart attack (as if all patients with heart attacks were cared for in the same way). Instead, the problem-solving question gives an outline of an *individual* – her age and family background, her mental state, her operation or diagnosis. The question is then worded something like this: 'Using a problem-solving approach, discuss the care required by Mrs Meredith during her first postoperative day.' Thus, the student is asked to devise the likely problems experienced by that individual patient, and the ways in which the nurse could help to alleviate those problems. This is quite different from those questions that treated all patients with cholecystectomy as having no individual differences.

The principal danger of this type of question is that it is possible for a student to provide a sound answer outlining, say, aspects of postoperative care, but one which nevertheless fails to mention any patient problems. Consequently, it will fail to answer the question as it is worded, and will gain few marks. (See the later section, 'How to fail').

To illustrate this, contrast these two answers:

1. Mrs Meredith was given an injection of pethidine, and her blood pressure and respirations were closely monitored. A vomit bowl and tissues were placed within easy reach. She was encouraged to sleep for the rest of the day.

2. In order to reduce her postoperative pain, Mrs Meredith was given an injection of pethidine. Because this drug can cause a fall in both blood pressure and respiration rate these were monitored closely. Mrs Meredith felt rather nauseated, so a vomit bowl and some tissues were placed on her locker. She had a drip in her right hand, so her locker was moved to her left side so that she could reach things easily. Mrs Meredith felt very tired after her anxious wait for her operation, and also because of the anaesthetic, and so she was encouraged to sleep for the rest of the day.

ACTIVITY

As a brief activity, look at answer number two and underline those words or phrases which seem to express a *problem* experienced by the patient. Can you understand how the second answer actually tackles the question, whereas the first, although accurately describing the care given, does not?

> Remember that a problem-solving question requires an answer that (a) suggests various patient problems, and (b) suggests solutions to them.

As you prepare for a nursing exam, it may be beneficial to think about the sort of patient problems that are likely to arise: preoperatively and postoperatively, and during emergency and routine admissions. Of course, some of these problems will vary according to the patient characteristics that are set out in the question itself, but others will remain the same. You will then have ready a partly prepared answer to this sort of problem-solving question in a number of common situations. This will save a good deal of time, rather than starting to devise your answer from scratch in the exam itself.

How to fail

Sadly, it is the case that a few students manage to fail examinations. Even though further attempts are allowed under most college regulations, it is probably wise not to tempt fate by waiting until your very last chance to succeed. Considering that exam questions are devised in order to *encourage* you to demonstrate your knowledge, and that the markers are looking for every opportunity to pass you, it is probably the case that you have to try hard in order to fail.

Here, then, are my suggestions for what you should do in order to fail your exam. To be rather more serious, here are some of the more frequent reasons for students to fail.

1. Probably the commonest reason for failure is **not to answer the question**. We saw earlier how this could be achieved in a question based on a problem-solving approach, but there are other situations where this can happen. You should read every word of the question in order to decide what it is the markers are wanting from you. You cannot rewrite the question, turning it into an 'everything-I-know-about-gallbladders' question.

   Thus, where a question requires you to relate a patient's clinical features to altered physiology, you must do exactly that. It is no good simply describing the clinical features presented by the patient.

   Where a question asks you to write your answer by referring to the activities of living (a feature of the popular Roper, Logan & Tierney model of nursing) this is what you must do. If you manage to describe the care of your given patients without mentioning any of the activities of living – like breathing, communicating, or maintaining body temperatures – your answer will gain few marks.

> Read and re-read the question. You cannot rewrite it to suit yourself. Each question has to be answered *as it is set.*

2. Another favourite method of failing exams is to **ignore the exam instructions**. I mentioned some of these earlier, such as choosing a certain number of questions

from specified sections of the paper. You can easily fail by answering too few questions – three, rather than the four you were asked to attempt. If you answer more than the required number of questions you won't necessarily fail, but you will have wasted a lot of time on that extra question that simply won't be marked.

3. Sometimes I have marked answers to nursing exams which contain **no reference to the course**. There is nothing in the answers to suggest the students have spent three years nursing. Instead, the answers consist of a superficial presentation of general knowledge. Often, exam instructions require students to refer in their answers to their own clinical experience. Where this is stipulated it should be followed. It is always good to read that a student has managed to see links between what he has carried out in the community or on the wards, and what he has learned in the lecture room.

4. **Inappropriate time management** is a well tried method of failing exams. The student concentrates on the exam questions she prefers, writing far more than is necessary for her first answer, only a little less for her second and third, but leaving 10 minutes for the fourth question, her least favourite. The very low mark she gains for the final answer will sometimes serve to pull down the average mark, leading to the award of a fail grade. I discuss the importance of managing time a little later. Incidentally, leaving sad little notes at the end of your paper – 'Sorry, I've run out of time' – does not earn you any marks, though it may make your examiner sad as he fails you.

5. **Superficial answers** don't earn many marks, especially when the question requires you to *discuss* a certain issue. This is often linked with point three above, for answers can consist simply of trite statements, based on general knowledge, and with no reference at all to the professional health care course that has been followed for 3 years, either its literature or its clinical experience. Answers include broad generalizations, and present the student's opinions as fact, with no reference to research to back them up. (One well-remembered answer, to a question on nutrition and health, included the breathtaking claim that black women ate too much because their menfolk preferred making love to fat women.)

   Where references are included in an answer, they should form part of the discussion. Names and dates sprinkled across the page do not impress markers, unless there is some attempt to incorporate them within the discussion. References should be relevant; sometimes I feel that the student knows a particular reference, has spent time and energy learning it by heart, and he is determined to include it in his answer whether it fits or not.

6. As with essays and projects, poor **grammar and spelling** in an exam do not lead to a fail. Neither do they enhance a student's work or a marker's overall impression of it. However, where a small percentage of marks is awarded for presentation – layout, spelling, grammar and handwriting – it seems a shame to throw them away. Unlike essays and projects written in your own time, you cannot use a word processor or typewriter in an exam (as far as I know), and so you have to rely on your handwriting. This is why I advised, in an earlier chapter, that those with problematic handwriting should take every opportunity to improve it before their final examination.

   Poor handwriting not only contributes to an initial poor impression, it also makes marking difficult, and it may serve to irritate your marker. A good-natured, benevolent marker may try more carefully to squeeze those important extra marks out of your work, than one who is annoyed and tired. This is *not* to say that poor writing will lead to a fail. However, writing that is completely illegible cannot be marked, and consequently will gain no marks.

WRITING FOR PUBLICATION

Appearances really do count, whether you are writing an exam answer or submitting a typescript to a publisher. A typescript that appears neat, with the correct margins and the minimum of alterations, and with grammar and spelling that are reasonably accurate, will be regarded more favourably by an editor. If your typescript requires a lot of editorial work before it can be accepted, an editor may come to the conclusion that it is not worth her while.

Revising for exams

Only you know how best to revise, just as you know what are the best conditions under which you can study. (You might like to reread those earlier pages which discussed personal preferences for studying – see Chapter 2.) Nevertheless, within your own constraints and preferences, the important word for effective revision is *planning*. Whether you have 1 or 3 hours a day available for revision, that time should be *planned*. Whether you intend to study throughout your days off or whether you're going to use them for relaxation, your study time needs to be *planned*.

Only planning can help you to overcome that sense of panic as you contemplate the great pile of notes you've collected throughout your course.

Revision will test the effectiveness with which you've organized your course notes. If you're reading this book right at the beginning of your course, decide now to organize your notes logically so as to make your future revision easier. It is not a good idea, for example, to stuff together in a ring binder all the notes relating to, say, Week 7 of your study block, whatever the topics covered. Instead, you may consider using dividers to separate subjects such as physiology, social policy, ethics and psychology.

Within those broad divisions, you can subdivide further. Under 'Physiology', for example, you might use different coloured notepaper for different systems of the body. During my nurse training, I used reporters' notebooks (those which are spiral bound at the top) to make rough notes during lectures. These were then transferred to A4 paper as soon as possible after the lecture, for inclusion in the appropriate ring binder. To these reorganized lecture notes on, say, myocardial infarction (heart attack) I added notes taken from various textbooks, including those on anatomy and physiology and nursing care. Later in my course, I was able to add notes made while working on a Coronary Care Unit, together with examples of ECGs (electrocardiographs) from patients who had suffered heart attacks.

My own nursing course was very much medically based, but in a current nursing curriculum you would gain notes from subjects like ethics, social policy, psychology and communication skills which could be associated with your clinical notes on myocardial infarction. One way of keeping tabs on relevant notes in other folders is to incorporate cross referencing throughout your notes. So, after your notes on the nursing care of a patient following a heart attack you could include references such as: 'See Ethics notes, p. 34' or 'See Social Policy notes, p. 14'.

Your revision will consist of more than reading each folder of notes through from beginning to end. If your revision timetable informs you that today you must revise the care of a patient with a heart attack, you know that your revision will take in all those cross references you've already built into your notes: anatomy and physiology, social policy, ethics, and communication skills. To revise your chosen subject, then, you'll be moving from folder to folder, following the links you've already forged during your course.

To revise is to revisit the knowledge already stored, but don't make the mistake of assuming that the only stored knowledge you've got from your course is in those

> Logical planning of your notes from the beginning of your course aids effective revision towards the end.

ring binders. There is probably far more knowledge inside your head (though you will probably dispute that as your exams get nearer). This stored knowledge is the result of your earlier struggles with the literature, with your clinical placements, and from lectures and seminars. Facts and discussions have passed through your brain en route for your notes. To revise, then, is to tap into that store of knowledge in your mind, as well as your folders.

If you can make your revision an *active* process you stand a better chance of securing important knowledge ready for the exams. By this I mean don't just read through notes, no matter how many times you can before the dreaded day arrives. Try and work at your notes by writing out major points, summarizing, jotting down fresh arguments, looking at a subject from different angles. By doing this you're putting your brain 'into gear', searching your mind for further insights beyond the brief notes in front of you on the page.

Sometimes it pays to revisit a given subject by reading the relevant section in a textbook you've not used before. (Incidentally, I would always recommend students not to rely on one text, but to use two or three.) It sometimes helps to discover another author's approach to a topic, perhaps examining it from a slightly different point of view.

Revising actively

Let's look at a subject suitable for revision, and see how we can make the revision process an active one, and thus more interesting and valuable: the care of an elderly patient with rheumatoid arthritis.

Whether you're a student therapist or nurse, it is likely that you will have notes about the sort of professional interventions which can assist such a client – physiotherapy of joints, medication, means of maintaining independence at home, for example. It is also likely that you'll have met at least one elderly patient with arthritis on a hospital ward, or in her own home, in your clinical circuit of experience.

You might begin your revision session, therefore, by searching your memory for details about a patient with rheumatoid arthritis for whom you've actually cared. Try and bring up an image of her face, and the way her affected joints looked. (For example, how did she pick up a cup to have a drink?) What drugs was she taking for pain? Did she go to the hospital pool for hydrotherapy and, if so, how much benefit did she derive from this? Did she use special cutlery at mealtimes? Ask yourself: what did *I* do for that patient?

You might try applying a problem-solving approach to the care of this remembered patient. What problems did she have or, if you can't recollect exactly, what problems would she be likely to have, given her diagnosis? You might think about problems such as:

- pain that keeps her awake at night
- tiredness during the day
- a poor appetite
- difficulty getting to the toilet in time
- a tendency to depression
- difficulty getting dressed and undressed.

There are bound to be many more problems you can think of.

You will see that you are already revising – revisiting – your knowledge about the given subject without as yet reading a single word of your notes. You're making your brain do the work (which is a very un-physiological way of putting it, but you'll know what I mean). You are tapping into the knowledge that's stored in your mind, even though, when faced with exams, it is usual for students to persuade themselves that they've remembered absolutely nothing. The image of a patient or client you've actually cared for is a very helpful 'releasing factor' for your stored

When faced with a question concerning a certain illness, try and remember a patient you've actually cared for who suffered from that same illness. Try and remember: 'How did I care for him?'

knowledge about the care and management of a similar patient, as specified in an exam question.

Having written down likely patient problems, now you might turn to your course notes about the nursing or therapeutic care of a patient with rheumatoid arthritis.

ACTIVITY

As well as nursing care, or care by therapists, for this patient, in what other sections of your stored notes might you also look for relevant information? Think about this before you look at my suggestions below.

One obvious place to look is your notes on human physiology, in order to revise the normal functioning of joints. Another is your notes on pathophysiology – what goes wrong in diseases like arthritis. Since the subject for revision is an elderly client, you may also have notes on the ageing process that would be of value. And if one of the patient problems you've listed is depression, this will guide you to another section of your notes, such as mental health problems and relevant communication skills. Another place to look is your notes on pharmacology, for details about the drugs your client could be taking. (Don't forget to read about the added danger of side effects from drugs when the patient is elderly.)

In revising the care of an elderly client with arthritis, you're using both your notes and your brain as a conjoined reference library, hunting through the pages (and the mental 'pages') for different collections of useful information. By changing the emphasis of your revision slightly, you can continue the *active* nature of your work; so, for example, you could think about the care of an elderly woman with arthritis on an acute ward (with an illness which may not be connected with her chronic condition). Or you could consider the care of such a patient at home, trying to live as independent a life as possible. What problems occur for the patient in either case? Is there additional information you need to look up? You might like to think, for instance, about the statutory and voluntary help that is available to clients in their own homes, and also about how well the acute wards you've worked on are geared towards coping with physically disabled patients.

Each time you alter the direction from which you study your chosen revision subject, your mind is brought into play in an active way, far more than if you are content merely to read through your notes from beginning to end. With the latter, you hope that constant repetition will help a few facts to 'stick', so that you can repeat them in your exam. With a more active process of revision, you are using

> Simply reading through your notes is boring and ineffective. The more active your revision can be the more you will enjoy it and the better you will be prepared for your exams.

ACTIVITY

This activity can be tried if you are some way into your course, and have accumulated both a fair amount of notes and some clinical experience.

Your teachers will supply you with both past exam papers and mock exam questions on which you can practise during the run up to the exams. Choosing two or three different exam questions, draw a diagram for each showing which sections of your notes you might study, and which areas of your clinical experience you might consider, in order to revise for them satisfactorily. I've done this as a guide in Figure 11.1, which illustrates the sources for revising a question relating to our familiar elderly client with rheumatoid arthritis.

You could try this activity, if you are at the beginning of your course, with a small group of colleagues. You'll already have some idea about the different subject areas contributing to your course, and this will guide your discussion. You may also be able to conjecture which clinical areas would prove useful.

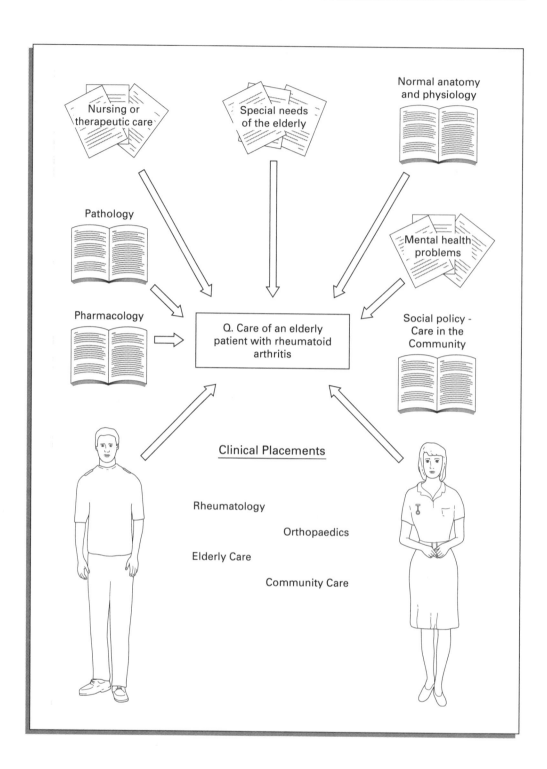

Figure 11.1
Sources for revision.
Subject: an elderly patient with
rheumatoid arthritis.

your notes (and your clinical and field recollections) far more thoroughly, sharpening your mind so that it can address more fully the questions that you are actually asked. This active revision also helps to draw strong links between practical experience (on the ward and in the community) and theoretical knowledge (derived from both lectures and textbooks). Such links, when demonstrated in an exam answer, can gain you further very useful marks.

When should revision begin?

Almost certainly you will hear of people who claim not to revise at all for exams, or who crammed for just 3 days beforehand. The trick is to pay no attention to such extravagant and unhelpful claims. You are in command of your own revision process, so it is you who will decide when to start – and when to stop.

For my own nursing final exams back in 1976, I started revising 6 months before the exam date . . . and gave up, bored to tears, 3 months later. This was clearly an inappropriate way of preparing for my exams.

The following is my tentative suggestion for an overview of a revision timetable. You should adapt it to suit your own needs and preferences:

- 12 weeks before exam – plan detailed timetable
- 11 weeks before exam – get notes into order
- 9 weeks before exam – start revising
- 3 days before exam – stop revising

Build into your timetable time for leisure. No one is going to give you any time off except yourself. It is difficult to study after coming off duty from a busy ward or community practice, so there is always the temptation to pile your revision onto your days off. It takes some courage to set aside one of those free days for you to enjoy, even though you will almost certainly feel guilty about doing so: 'Why am I shopping when I should be revising?' you'll ask yourself. Try and be firm. Tell yourself you deserve, you *need*, time for relaxation.

I would never recommend last minute cramming just before an exam. Certainly you shouldn't open your books or your notes on the morning of the exam itself. My advice would be to reward yourself with the 3 days leading up to the exam as a time for relaxation, but this may be too long a time for your conscience to allow you. Can you and your conscience settle for just 1 day free prior to the exam?

(You may like to reread the section called 'Don't kid yourself' in Chapter 2. Its relevance to revision lies with using your time wisely by actually timing the period you set aside for revision, rather than relying on the gut feeling that 'I must have been working for *hours*!' Also reread my comments in 'Managing your time' about using a system of rewards for accomplishing revision.)

Practising writing exam answers

As part of your revision process, try and write practice answers to either past exam papers or the mock papers provided by your teacher – always supposing that the exam's format hasn't changed. You may find it useful to write, say, one full answer each week, and two or three answers in note form. You must, however, have your personal tutor's agreement to mark your efforts and, more important than a mark or grade, to provide you with full comments. Bear in mind that your tutor may well have many more students' work to mark in the weeks leading up to an exam – on top of her usual teaching and preparation – so you should be prepared to expect a certain time lapse between handing in your script and getting it back with her advice.

What is most important is that the answers you write are completed **within the correct time limit** for your approaching exam. There is little point in lavishing an hour on one answer when in the exam itself you will have only 45 minutes per question. When you write answers in note form, you would do well to reduce the amount of time you allow yourself appropriately – say, from 45 minutes to 15.

Concentrate not just on getting words down on paper, but on *planning* each answer you write. In your revision, and in the exam itself, you should certainly set aside some time for planning. If each question merits 45 minutes, then it is probably reasonable to allocate 8 to 10 minutes to its planning. This will mean that your answer, when you come to write it, will move ahead smoothly and logically, instead of being simply a jumble of ideas, shoved down on the paper as they occur to you.

Now, this takes courage. It takes courage on your part to sit in an exam room *not* scribbling furiously as all those around you seem to be doing. There is a strong temptation to use every minute of the exam to get words down on paper. However, you really do *save* time by utilizing it wisely. Spending 10 minutes planning your answer will, I am convinced, help you to write a better answer with consequent higher marks. An answer which is broken up into headings, subheadings, and paragraphs (as with any essay you're asked to write at college) is much easier to follow by the examiner, and therefore easier to mark, than one that follows a sort of 'flow of consciousness' model.

Planning an answer tends to help you actually answer the question as it is written. Writing down ideas immediately they occur to you, conversely, will risk *not* answering the examiners' question, but instead produce one of those 'all-I-know-about' answers I've mentioned before.

Planning also helps you direct your thoughts, in a specific way, towards the goal of a logical answer. It helps you avoid those meaningless phrases that seem so commonly to occur in exam answers which are unplanned. Such phrases include:

- all nursing care
- routine observations
- maintain the patient's airway.

The examiner of a nursing exam will want you to provide details about the nursing care you deliver, so 'all nursing care' tells her nothing about your understanding of the given patient's needs.

'Routine observations' tells the marker nothing about your level of knowledge regarding such nursing interventions. Do you actually know what they are, or why they are done, or how often? (Should nursing observations, made on an individualized basis, ever be regarded as 'routine'?)

It is often an excellent idea to 'maintain the patient's airway' – for example, during an epileptic fit – but this phrase doesn't tell us *how* the nurse achieves this. There are some methods of trying to maintain the patient's airway during a fit that would be considered dangerous for the nurse, such as inserting her fingers into the patient's mouth. The examiner wants details concerning the position in which the patient is placed, the type of airway that might be used, or whether oxygen is called for or not.

Another dangerous word to use when describing care is 'regularly': 'The patient's blood pressure was recorded regularly.' Fine – but once a year for the next 5 years is regular; is this what you mean? Instead, the marker needs to know whether you consider this particular patient's blood pressure should be recorded every 2 hours, or every 15 minutes.

It is lack of initial planning that leads to a meandering answer with imprecise phrases – and ultimately to a low mark.

My final point about writing practice answers for an exam is that I don't believe it is sensible to 'question spot'. By this I mean studying your college's recent past papers, noting that certain topics haven't appeared, and consequently revising especially for them in the belief that they'll come up next time. You may be lucky, but you are risking a great deal. To note that the subject of myocardial infarction, for example, occurred in the previous paper, doesn't mean that you can safely assume it won't be there next time. It is such an important nursing subject that it could well appear but with a somewhat different emphasis.

However, you may feel able to leave certain topics out of your revision plans. For example, if your clinical nursing experience included the Ear, Nose and Throat ward, rather than ophthalmology, you may sensibly omit the latter from your revision, since you have no relevant clinical experience on which to 'hang' your theoretical knowledge gained from lectures and textbooks.

> More planning . . . less wasted time . . . more marks.

ACTIVITY

How to avoid waffle

It occasionally happened that some of my students had difficulty in limiting the amount they wrote in mock answers, and also in planning their answers around paragraphs, with one paragraph per idea. I tried to devise a practice method that physically constrained the amount they could write on a given topic, and which also helped them plan their answers. This system may be useful for you, too, so I include it here.

Imagine that you are in my office, with your pen and A4 pad ready. Now I'm going to guide you through each step of the practice.

Let's take as a revision topic, 'Care of the breathless patient following operation'. (Because I'm restricting this activity to just four aspects of care, the exact wording of the exam question is less important.)

First I ask you to write down, using either **single words** or **short phrases**, a number of nursing interventions relating to the given topic. Four of these interventions you write are:

1. oxygen
2. position in bed
3. chest physiotherapy
4. pain relief.

Now, for each of these, you are next asked to write **one brief explanatory sentence**, one that summarizes the care given. (I used to tell my students they were restricted to two lines of an A4 pad for each sentence.) Choosing points two and four above, you might write:

2. The patient is sat up in bed, well supported by pillows.
4. The patient is kept free of pain by giving the prescribed analgesia.

After checking the sentences you've written, I explain the next stage of the practice. This involves turning each **sentence** into a **paragraph**, so that you will end up with about four or five paragraphs of reasonably detailed prose. In order to restrict the amount you can write (thus hoping to avoid waffle), a panel or boundary line is drawn on your notepad, one panel for each paragraph, and each enclosing only about 7 lines. Each panel could begin with a subheading, perhaps using the single words or brief phrases obtained in stage one of the process.

For the final stage, you are asked to write a brief introduction and an equally brief conclusion to your set of paragraphs, perhaps restricting each to about five lines.

It helps, I think, if you now read out the entire essay, both for my comments and so that you are able to appreciate how it flows, and how the various elements of nursing care are confined to their own paragraphs. The final version is a much better planned essay than one that would emerge from an unplanned brainstorming session.

Look after yourself – and each other

I would guess that sitting exams is perhaps the most stressful assessment procedure through which colleges put their students. It concerns me greatly that, while an element of stress is useful for motivating all of us to work harder and with greater concentration, for some students stress can increase to unhealthy and dangerous levels. It is when revising for exams that students should particularly keep an eye out for colleagues who appear to be overly anxious, or who are attempting to cope with their stress in an unhealthy way.

No assessment strategy should lead, in my view, to its students seeking tranquillizers from their doctors, or sedation to help them sleep at night. Neither should students find themselves seeking solace in increasing amounts of alcohol. Sharing a drink with your friends after an evening's hard labour over your notes and textbooks is one thing; sitting alone in your room with no other company but cans of lager is quite another.

> While you're revising, keep an eye on your friends as well as your books. Look after your own health, and look after each other during this stressful time.

I suggested earlier that you should insist that part of your time be set aside for relaxation, and I repeat that advice here. Any form of relaxation which gets you away from your books, your room, and your library, can be no bad thing. Go jogging with friends, or indulge in some hard games of squash, or, as I did when revising for university exams, climb mountains. Whatever you choose, exercise and fresh air, good company and the expenditure of large amounts of physical energy, should play their part in keeping you healthy.

Easy though it is for me to give you advice, make sure you maintain a proper balanced diet throughout your revision, and that you allow yourself plenty of time for sleep. You cannot survive prolonged periods of revision on a regime of black coffee, cigarettes, and late nights. If you possibly can, avoid tablets that either calm you down or pick you up. Conversely, if you feel you simply aren't coping, go to your doctor straight away, and seek the help of your personal tutor and your friends. Don't suffer in isolation and silence.

The great day arrives

On the day of the exam itself, *don't* look at your books and notes. You should instead concentrate on packing your bag with the appropriate pens, pencils, erasers, and refills. Take dictionaries with you if they're allowed. Most examination boards allow students to take drinks and food into the exam room, but you should avoid unpacking sandwiches with much rustling of paper wrappings, or setting up a primus stove to brew tea. In today's more humane climate, students are permitted to empty their bladders during the exam (I mean, in the appropriate place) unlike my day when we had no choice but to cross our legs or give up the exam halfway through. (Neither was food allowed then, but the long sleeves of our academic gowns – which had to be worn to gain entry to the exam room – were ideal for concealing large bars of chocolate.)

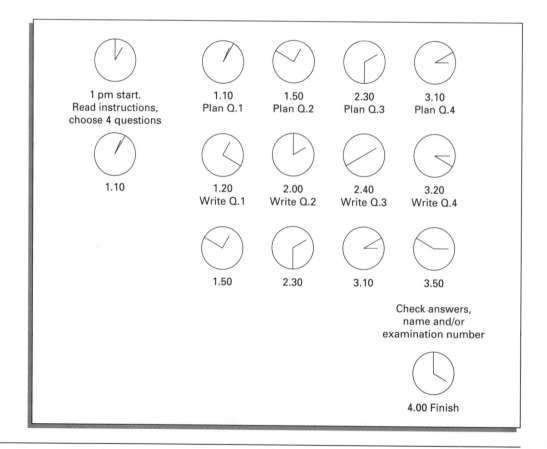

Figure 11.2
Planning and writing times for a 3-hour session.

Before you turn over the question paper, you will already know how many questions you have to attempt, and how much time you should spend on each. Tell yourself once again that you *will* spend a few minutes reading the exam instructions at the head of the paper, that you *will* read each question thoroughly, and that you will *plan* each answer carefully. If you prefer, quickly draw up a diagram that gives you the appropriate times for each question, both planning and writing (as in Figure 11.2).

After making your choice of questions you're going to attempt, underline their key words. Don't, above all, rewrite your question. You will gain marks only for answering the question **as it is written**. It's a good idea, 10 minutes into your answer, to look back at the question again. Ask yourself: 'Am I answering it, or my own version of it?'

Don't allow panic to begin, especially when your initial glance over the questions in front of you persuades you that you can't possibly answer any of them. Of course you can! You've spent 3 years working towards this moment; you have 3 years of studying, and working in the clinical and fieldwork areas, to help you jump this particular hurdle. A little time studying a question that at first seems beyond you, reveals that actually it's all about the admission of a patient for a planned operation, or about terminal care, or about chest physiotherapy to someone on an intensive care unit.

You may have your own preferred method of reducing anxiety at such times, such as concentrating on your breathing, and gradually slowing down your respiration rate. Or you may choose to repeat a short prayer or mantra in your mind for just a few minutes. Above all, try and regard that exam paper in front of your as an invitation to show off your knowledge. It's not there to trip you up; it hasn't been set by fiends who are anxious to fail you and half your student group too. It consists of carefully worded problems, based on a health care setting that you have been studying for 3 years, which invite you to solve them.

Above all, have faith in your own ability to answer those questions well, and in your marker's ability to find all the marks you could possibly need to pass.

And afterwards

At the end of the exam, hand your paper in to the invigilator, **and walk away**. Don't indulge in frantic postmortem discussions outside the exam room with your colleagues, in which you realize what you omitted from Question 3, and how you got the wrong end of the stick in Question 7. There is nothing more you can do to change your fate, except wait for the day of the results.

In the meantime, continue to look after yourself and your colleagues. This *is* an anxious and difficult period with which to cope, and there might well be certain friends who particularly need your support. Go out together, get a little merry together, and stick together. You are all student nurses and therapists so if *you* can't look after each other, who else can?

REFERENCE
Collins English Dictionary 3rd edn 1991 Harper Collins, Glasgow

N o t e s

12 Continuing assessment in the clinical area

Key topics

- ■ The terminology of clinical supervision
- ■ Working under supervision in the clinical area
- ■ Undergoing clinical assessment
- ■ The place of clinical assessment within the overall assessment process

Much of this book has been concerned with written assessments for health care students. This is not, however, to undervalue the part played by clinical assessments in the student's personal and professional development. Indeed, for professions such as nursing, physiotherapy, and occupational therapy, it is highly appropriate that the hands-on skills of future registered practitioners should be tested, and rigorously.

Yet how should such testing be carried out, and by whom? At the beginning of this book, I described how, in my own nurse training, bed making skills were tested by means of an essay. Of course logistically, it was probably easier for the tutor to mark 32 essays than to watch 32 students making 32 beds. Nevertheless, observing a student carrying out client care would seem to be a surer method of assessing his practical skills than reading his essay describing those skills.

One problem with writing about the care that should be given by a nurse or therapist, is that the written description of care might not reflect the student's ability or intention to provide it. Just because he *writes* that he would carefully smooth out the creases in the bottom sheet, doesn't mean that he will actually *do* this in the frantic bustle of a surgical ward.

Some exam papers attempt to get close to the clinical or field situation by requiring students to write essays discussing the care of profiled clients – an elderly woman following hernia repair; a middle-aged man with a heart attack. Even so, however closely examiners link such questions to the community or to hospital wards, they do not really test the student's clinical skills. Again, because I write in an essay that I will apply certain listening skills when helping a severely depressed client, it does not follow that, in the clinical situation, I am capable of deploying those skills. (To describe many communication skills is probably far easier than performing them.)

Essays and examinations test a student's knowledge and understanding, as well as her ability to work within time constraints, and to seek out, marshal, and present relevant material. However, to test a student's ability to empathize with a patient in pain, or a client frustrated by his inability to dress himself, she must be observed in the clinical situation, in her interactions with her patient or client.

This is easier to state than to carry out. A senior physiotherapist might observe her student correctly placing his hands on the patient's chest in order to carry out breathing exercises. So far so good. But how is this practical procedure to be judged? Are marks awarded for the volume of sputum expectorated by the patient? For the lack of broken ribs at the end of the procedure? And how will the student's manner be judged? It is perhaps easy to note that he is *either* empathic and gentle, *or* off-hand and unsympathetic, but it is less easy to judge intervening standards.

In order for a student to be assessed practically on a ward or in a community setting, he must have the opportunity first to practise those skills on which he is to be assessed. He needs to know clearly *when* he is to be assessed, *by whom*, and *what* aspects of care will be assessed.

Working under supervision

Before Project 2000 changed the face of nurse education in Britain, it is probably true to say that student nurses formed the major part of the nursing workforce in training hospitals, or at least on training wards. It was quite common, for example, for a morning shift on a busy ward to be staffed by just one trained nurse, with four or five students. Trained nurse supervision was, for obvious reasons, minimal. Often it would consist of instructions concerning patient care given during the report at the beginning of the shift, followed by the students reporting back to the nurse in charge at the end of the shift. Meanwhile the trained nurse's time may well have been taken up with doctors' rounds, answering telephone enquiries, and caring for the most severely ill patients.

Junior students learned most of all by working with more senior students. There was no question of working with a named supervising registered nurse. This situation was less likely to occur with student physiotherapists and occupational therapists, where often one student would work alongside a trained practitioner.

With Project 2000 the question of monitoring the development of student nurses' practical skills was tackled vigorously. No longer was it deemed acceptable for students to be thrown in at the deep end, to sink or swim. Colleges of nursing were required to run preparation programmes for registered nurses who were to supervise students. College curricula had to state how often these supervisors must work alongside their students.

Problems of definition

The title of these supervisors seemed to cause great confusion, and articles in the nursing press argued for and against terms such as mentor, preceptor, supervisor, facilitator, and several more. Now, it is probably more important for you, as a relatively new student approaching your first clinical placement, to know the name given by *your* college to *your* supervisor, rather than to follow the intricacies of the debate. But the following brief account of the literary discussion might explain why different courses use different supervisory titles.

The term perhaps most commonly applied to the supervising role undertaken by trained nurses was **mentor**. This word, Armitage & Burnard explain (1991), first arose in USA business schools, and from there spread to American colleges of nursing. It then crossed the Atlantic without, however, the benefit of clear definition. 'Mentor' was somewhat loosely taken to mean an experienced nurse whose job it was to look after and guide less experienced nurses.

In mental health nursing, Morris et al (1988) describe four possible functions of the mentor: role model, facilitator, supervisor, and assessor. Anforth (1992) is clear, though, that 'mentor' is not synonymous with 'assessor'. A senior nurse, she writes, cannot be expected one day to guide and befriend (the mentoring role) and the next to assess. By contrast, Morris et al assert that 'the mentor is the obvious candidate to be the learner's assessor' (p. 26). Guidelines from the English National Board (ENB) in 1988 proved to be less clear than desired, though they did state that 'it is important that the students know which role the person is occupying at any given time' (i.e. mentor or assessor). So it seemed to be the ENB view that one experienced nurse could be *both* mentor *and* assessor.

After struggling for 3 years with the ENB guidelines Barlow, a director of nurse education, no less, threw them aside and concluded that the mentor role is best adopted by a student's personal tutor (Barlow 1991). However, she fails to address the possible problem of a student facing a disciplinary hearing. How can a tutor be an effective mentor (friend, guide, role model) if he may one day be part of a disciplinary panel that could terminate his student's nurse training? I wonder, too, how credible a role model a nurse tutor can be in the clinical situation. Surely an experienced ward-based nurse is better placed to be a role model for a student working on a ward?

To complicate matters further, Armitage & Burnard (1991) argue persuasively that the mentor role is incompatible with the concept of student nurse as autonomous adult learner. Rather, students should receive clinical supervision from a *preceptor*, who acts as guide and role model, helping them to learn 'on the job'. However, Morton-Cooper & Palmer (1993), in their 'Glossary of Support Roles', reserve the term 'preceptor' for an experienced practitioner, with responsibility for her own client group, who acts as guide, teacher and supervisor to a *newly qualified nurse*, midwife, or health visitor.

Most authors seem to agree that it is necessary for a relationship to develop between mentor and student, and for this reason, write Morris et al (ibid.), no less than 3 months with the same mentor is required. The average period of time, in their mental health setting, for a student to stay with the same mentor is 6 months. Barlow is more dismissive, stating that 'the hierarchical structure of nursing in the UK mitigates against the type of relationship normally found between mentor and protégé' (ibid. p. 53). Presumably this same structure would rule out autonomous adult learning, too.

There is general agreement that prospective mentors require a period of special training for their role. However, this varies somewhat dramatically between a half-day workshop (Anforth 1992) and a week (Morris et al 1988).

As a comparatively new student nurse, facing your first ward-based experience, you may now be a little confused. Just who is going to be supervising you on the ward – personal tutor, ward tutor, mentor (whatever that means), preceptor, facilitator . . . or a couple of your own colleagues?

It is unlikely to be the latter, though you will certainly learn much in discussion with them in your shared time off duty, or in group evaluations of clinical experience. One of your main tasks at the beginning of your ward placement is to obtain a clear statement from your college about the level and frequency of clinical supervision you are to receive, and from whom. I would suggest that it is less important what label is hung around the neck of your supervisor, and more important to discover who she is, what her role is, and how often you can expect to work with her.

> Find out who will be your ward or community supervisor, and how often you should work with her.

If your college uses the terms 'mentor' or 'preceptor', it is important for you to ascertain what *your* college means by them, for that is what will affect your clinical supervision. 'Mentor' might be the name given to your supervisor on each of your allocated wards. Now if you spend only, say, 10 weeks on a ward, both your days off duty and your mentor's days off duty (to say nothing of sickness, holidays and night shifts) may mean there is very little time for this special mentor–student relationship to develop. You will be lucky if you enjoy more than, on average, one day's direct supervision per week. You should also ascertain, therefore, who will undertake your clinical supervision in your ward mentor's absence.

On the other hand, your college may reserve the term 'mentor' for an experienced nurse who occupies a supervisory role somewhere between your personal tutor and the supervisor given to you on each of your wards. For example, you may be allocated a mentor during your Common Foundation Programme in nursing, and another during your Branch Programme, while you keep the same personal tutor for the whole 3 years of your course. In this situation, both your tutor and your mentor will have an input to the way in which your clinical learning is assessed.

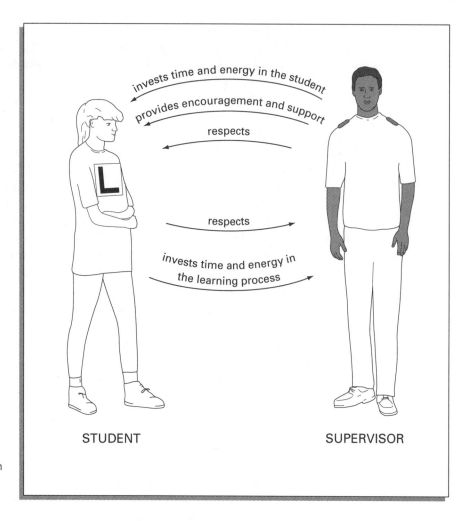

invests time and energy in the student

provides encouragement and support

respects

respects

invests time and energy in
the learning process

STUDENT   SUPERVISOR

Figure 12.1
Supervisor and student roles –
respect for each other, and dual
investment of time and energy. Each
individual learns from the other.

For the rest of this chapter, however, I will steer well clear of the debate by using the term 'supervisor' for an experienced registered nurse or therapist, who works with you and guides you through your clinical or field placements. I have tried to show important features of the student/supervisor relationship in Figure 12.1. While some of the literature states that the student respects or looks up to his supervisor, I've suggested in the figure that such respect is a two-way process. A supervisor who holds her student(s) in high regard is likely to be the recipient of equally high regard.

It is so important for you to discover your own college's definition of the supervisory terms they use, such as 'mentor' and 'preceptor', that it is worth repeating the point I made earlier in the form of an Activity.

ACTIVITY

Before starting your clinical and field placements, find out which term your college uses to refer to the supervisor(s) who will act as your guide and role model there. Clarify your college's requirements for these helpers – how often they should work with you each week, and what exactly their helping role will include. Are there 'deputy' supervisors who will help you when your principal supervisor is away from the ward? Will there be separate assessors, or will your practical assessments be carried out by your ward supervisor? What are the responsibilities of your personal tutor and ward tutors during your clinical placements? What part will they play in your clinical assessments?

You, too, will have an important role to play in your personal and professional development, while on the wards and in the community. *Your* role will be a leading one – assessing (with help) the progress you've made so far in your course, identifying any possible areas of weakness, and planning the best ways in which to meet the learning outcomes or objectives set down for you by the college, and those you've drawn up for yourself.

Incidentally, in assessing your own progress, don't be afraid to pat yourself on the back for achieving your learning outcomes. It is my experience that many students are more negative about their progress than are their appointed assessors, certainly more than their progress merits. Praise yourself from time to time.

Planned learning in the clinical areas

Working effectively in the clinical areas will help you achieve the learning outcomes established by your college curriculum. For this reason, I'm going to spend some time discussing ways in which you can *plan* your practical work, just as you might plan an essay or care study.

It is possible, I suppose, to work for 10 weeks or so on your allocated ward, in the hope that you will collide with certain useful learning opportunities. You might, for example, be nearby when staff nurse admits a patient who is severely ill. It would seem more sensible, however, and will make your experience far more interesting, to plan your learning from the very beginning of your allocation. Learning outcomes, drawn up by yourself, your supervisor, and tutor, will encourage you to seek out learning opportunities. Learning contracts can play a useful part in meeting those outcomes. Maintaining a learning log will help you respond positively and thoughtfully to the events that occur on your ward.

> It is as important to plan your clinical and field learning as it is to plan an essay.

1. Looking for learning opportunities

A hospital ward is a community rich in learning opportunities, not just for students like yourself, but for its trained nurses and therapists too. When caring for patients, you will find that you never stop learning. Human physiology gleaned from a textbook begins to come alive when you observe the clinical features of the patient in front of you. Here is an elderly woman, Mrs Carter, who appears pale and lethargic. Every movement she makes seems to tire her. It is almost too much for her to wash her hands and face. Her mouth is sore, she tells you, and she has no appetite. At home she ate very little, too, because she couldn't be bothered to shop or cook.

Your supervisor tells you that Mrs Carter's haemoglobin level is greatly reduced, probably because of a chronically poor diet since her husband died. You remember what your physiology text informed you about the function of red cells and haemoglobin. (Can you remember the normal adult female red cell count and haemoglobin level?) You begin to realize that, if you know what is the normal function of red blood cells, you can understand what might happen, clinically, if there aren't enough of them, or if their haemoglobin level is reduced. The patient's obvious lethargy now begins to make sense.

Your supervisor encourages you to sit and talk with Mrs Carter for a while: 'Ask her about the sort of meals she cooked for herself at home. Oh yes, and how far she lives from the shops, too.'

The ensuing conversation with your patient is more than a nice chat. Instead, it turns into both a *learning experience* for you and a *patient assessment*, because the information you gain is helpful in forming an accurate overall picture of Mrs Carter, and drawing up a successful care plan for her.

Staff nurse tells you Mrs Carter has been admitted in order to have a blood transfusion. 'Now,' he asks you, 'what did you learn about blood groups in college', and what observations will you make on Mrs Carter while she's having her transfusion?'

> Form the habit of making brief (but confidential) notes about your patients, and resolve to read about both their condition and their care when you get home from the ward.

Can you see, just from this simple example, how your learning-as-theory in college comes to the assistance of your learning-in-practice on the ward? Your supervisor has, rightly, prompted you to forge links between what you learned from textbooks and what you're currently learning from the patient in front of you. He might also ask you to suggest ways in which the patient's management could continue when she is discharged.

Patients are probably the finest learning resource for students on a health care course. But there are others.

2. Looking for additional learning resources

It is likely that the ward to which you've been allocated will have a collection of textbooks relevant to its own speciality. These may take you further than the more general texts you've purchased for yourself. One or two of these books may be loaned to you by the ward manager, or you may be given a certain amount of study time during your allocation to read them and make notes.

Often, wards maintain folders of useful information – articles from professional journals, research reports, brochures from drug and equipment companies. These can be an excellent source of up to date information, since articles usually can be published far more quickly than large textbooks.

ACTIVITY

Create your own information folder for subjects that interest you. In it include articles from professional journals, notes on drugs, and brochures on aids and equipment.

A patient's notes and X-rays, used appropriately and with careful supervision, are excellent sources of information. Remember that what you are reading is *confidential*. It sometimes happens that highly personal material is held in medical notes, such as someone's HIV status or a termination of pregnancy a long time ago. Supervision is important in order to steer you away from distant and complex areas of a patient's medical history, guiding you instead toward information that is more relevant to her present admission to hospital.

X-rays should be examined with the assistance of someone who understands them – and understanding takes time to develop. At first it may be that all you can spot are obvious bony features such as ribs and pelvis. Eventually, and with practice, you may be able to make out features such as gas within a loop of bowel, or a partially collapsed lung.

Other ward resources include members of the health care team who can provide a different slant on your patient's condition and management. His difficulties with mobilization may be explained by the physiotherapist who helps him exercise each morning. His apparent lack of appetite at mealtimes may be explained by the occupational therapist, who shows you how his reduced manual dexterity can be overcome with specially designed cutlery. A student physiotherapist may ask a trained nurse about the patient's pain control, in order to assess the best time for carrying out his breathing exercises.

It is usually the case that professionals are eager to pass on information to enquiring students. There is, however, a right time and a wrong time to ask questions.

3. Asking questions

I well remember as a staff nurse being asked, by a student new to the ward, whether the patient I was with wanted porridge or cereal for next day's breakfast. This would not have been so bad had the patient not been suffering a cardiac arrest at the time, and I was somewhat occupied with carrying out external cardiac massage.

Ward emergencies are not the best time for asking questions, unless to seek clarification about something you've been asked to do. It is during emergencies such as a cardiac arrest that trained staff understandably concentrate on the patient's immediate needs, rather than the student's.

When I worked on a coronary care unit (CCU) I tried to include our student nurses in cardiac resuscitation, with each staff nurse 'adopting' a student – one working with the anaesthetist, for instance, and another with the staff nurse drawing up cardiac drugs. I might then ask a student to jot down what drugs we were using, and the times they were injected. This important information could then be transferred to the patient's medical notes after the emergency was over. *Then* came the time when questions could appropriately be asked – why was that drug given, why didn't they use the defibrillator, and so on.

Unfortunately, during emergencies like a cardiac arrest, tempers can sometimes fray, and staff snap at each other. A student may seem too slow in fetching something, like a drip stand or some fresh syringes, and thus earns for himself some unflattering comments. The best professional will afterwards explain why she reacted as she did and, if appropriate, apologize. Also, the student's slowness should be examined, in a calmer atmosphere, in order to see if something can be learned from events. It is inadmissible, in my opinion, for a trained nurse to shout at a student who, in an emergency, is working too slowly, when he has not previously been shown how to do the required procedure. Save your questions until the atmosphere seems a little less strained, or quietly ask someone not so immediately involved in the action.

If you are asked to fetch a piece of equipment and you don't know what it is, or where it is kept, don't hesitate: tell the person. It is *not* your fault if you have never been shown the equipment or its hiding place.

4. Skills and microskills

Can you remember the first time you were shown how to use a computer? Perhaps your experience was similar to mine. The 'expert' sat in front of the machine and, while he delivered a long string of instructions (containing words I'd never heard before) his fingers rattled busily over the keyboard. And that was my tuition, after which I was expected to know how to use the wretched machine for myself.

In health care, many of the jobs we do are of a highly complex nature. This is why, for example, when learning communication skills, you have probably practised 'microskills' – small parts of the whole process of communicating.

ACTIVITY

Have you covered the important subject of 'Listening' in your communication skills classes yet? If so, try and remember how many facets there are to effective listening. Just to start you off, here is one:

● positioning yourself in relation to the client or patient.

Admitting and assessing a new patient to the ward is an immensely complex procedure. From the manner in which you greet your patient he will form an initial impression of the ward he is entering. From your detailed patient assessment you will derive important aspects of care, such as appropriate nursing observations to make.

Your supervisor would not expect you to admit and assess a patient on your first ward experience. Indeed, I would suggest that such a responsible procedure (or rather, a set of procedures) should be reserved for third year students. Even one element of patient assessment – taking his blood pressure – is a complex skill that can be broken down into several microskills. What is the best way of teaching a student to take someone's blood pressure? Like the computer expert I described earlier, I suppose your supervisor could demonstrate the whole thing from start to finish, then hand you the equipment (and someone's arm) and tell you to have a go yourself. There is a better way, however.

This is to demonstrate each separate part of the procedure and, after each demonstration, ask the student to practise it – just that one part. So, these individual microskills might include:

- positioning the sphygmomanometer (the blood pressure machine containing the mercury column) at the right level in relation to the patient
- positioning the earpieces of the stethoscope correctly and comfortably
- finding the correct spot on the patient's arm (or the arm of your colleague on whom you're practising) for placing the stethoscope membrane
- manipulating the screw valve, both to close it off and to let out air very gradually
- squeezing the rubber bulb while controlling the screw valve
- observing the falling mercury as you let air out of the cuff gradually.

I am sure there will be several more microskills you could include here, to say nothing about recognizing and knowing the significance of the various sounds that you hear through the stethoscope.

Interestingly, Morris et al (1988) describe one of the functions of their 1-week mentors' course as helping trained nurses (as potential mentors) to break down some of the skills they use every day into smaller 'microcompetencies', that could then be taught separately to their students. In this way, they write, acting as a role model becomes more than simply being observed by the student as they perform whole tasks.

I've chosen taking blood pressures as an example because, from my experience, students can find this a very daunting task. Sometimes students cannot initially hear anything through the stethoscope, and they become upset because they feel that in some way they have 'failed', both themselves and their patients.

As trained nurses, we have to remember that the jobs we do daily almost automatically can prove to be frightening and near-impossible for students fresh to the wards. A task such as giving an intramuscular injection can be particularly frightening because it carries with it the possibility of doing the patient harm, or hurting him. Giving injections, just like recording blood pressures, can be divided into microskills (or microcompetencies, as Morris et al call them) which should be practised separately. I would suggest the following programme of progress:

> Complex practical skills are best practised initially as a number of separate microskills, before being reassembled and practised together.

Practical skills – giving an intramuscular injection
- being with supervisor and observing whole task
- breaking down task into component microskills
- separate microskill practice under supervision
- whole task practice under supervision
- follow up discussion with supervisor, and perhaps with ward tutor – linking practical skill with theory
- continue practising whole task, but seeking help if needed
- assessment
- continue practising whole task.

This programme could, I think, be applied to many other tasks in the clinical setting. Note how *assessment* comes towards the end of the programme, when both student and supervisor feel the whole task has been practised sufficiently often. Using the examples of giving an injection or taking a blood pressure, these could play their part in the assessed total care of one patient for a morning or afternoon.

5. Using a learning contract

Learning contracts can be drawn up between tutor and student, and supervisor and student. They are a way of making formal promises both of learning effort and tutor help. They include details about *what* is to be achieved or performed, by *whom*, and *when*.

Contracts can be written at the suggestion of the student as well as the tutor and supervisor, so they should not be regarded as something always imposed on the student from on high. For example, in a discussion with her supervisor at the end of a ward shift, a student might say this:

■ *'I'm unhappy about giving out drugs to those patients we've been looking after today. Several of the medicines were new to me, and I don't know about their proper dosages or side effects. If I do some reading over my days off, will you go through the notes I make with me?'*

The student can be more challenging, if she feels this is appropriate to her situation:

■ *'When we gave out those drugs this morning, you didn't say anything about what they were for, or what their side effects were. Is that because you expected me to know already? It would be really helpful if you could tell me about the medicines we give out in future.'*

There is nothing wrong with asking for instruction!

A learning contract can be something agreed verbally or, preferably I think, in writing between two people. It's rather like making a bargain with someone:

● I agree to carry out X
● if you agree to do Y
● within the time span Z.

So the student above, unsure about the medicine she's witnessed being given to her patients, might suggest the following contract:

● By 12th September, I shall have read the chapter in Hopkins on antibiotics. I'll have written notes on what I've read, and I will bring them to the ward for my supervisor to see.

The student's supervisor adds the following:

● On 12th September I agree to meet Sandra in order to discuss the most important antibiotics we use on this ward. I shall have prepared a short list of the commonest drugs, their adult dosages, and their side effects, and I shall read and make comments on the notes Sandra has made.
● I agree in future to provide verbal information to Sandra whenever we give out medicines to our patients.
● I agree to ask Sandra questions relating to the drugs we gave out during our previous duties together.

That last sentence takes Sandra a little by surprise. It's a great idea, of course, but . . . So Sandra adds the following to her side of the contract:

● I agree to make a note of the unfamiliar drugs we give to our patients. I will then read about them in Hopkins when I get off duty, and I agree to be asked questions about them during our next duty together.

This contract between supervisor and student is formal in its wording, but it is also flexible, in that additions can be made to its terms. It sets out exactly what each person can expect of the other, and what each must do herself. It states *what* each has to do, and *when*, and remains as a written witness of the bargain struck between the people concerned. It can then be consulted by either party if disagreement arises.

Learning contracts can be employed in the classroom, as well as in the clinical or field areas. Contracts are particularly useful in tutorials, when both tutor and students state clearly what each can expect of the other. Drawing up contracts reflects very much the same positive regard each party has for the other as was shown in Figure 12.1.

6. Keeping a learning log

Captains of ships maintain logs of the voyages they make, detailing speed, weather conditions, and ports of call. Students entering clinical areas for the first time are themselves undertaking a voyage – a voyage of discovery. For them, keeping a log can be highly valuable.

In any new job, maintaining a learning log (or learning diary) can help you work more self-critically. You look more carefully at events that occur, as you describe them in your log, and think more critically about how you might respond to them.

I found a learning diary particularly useful during my practical placement as a tutor student, since I had gone straight from working as a charge nurse on the wards to attending a tutors' course, with no intervening period as an unqualified tutor (Goodall 1985). Each experience – teaching a large class, conducting a small-group seminar, interviewing applicants for nurse training, writing lesson plans – was thus entirely new, and I needed a means by which I could reflect after each event.

It is fairly easy for a log to become a simple statement of what happened: 'Got up, had breakfast, went to work, did a bedbath . . .' Such a diary is of little use either reading it in retrospect or as you are actually writing it. For example, read what Simon, a student nurse, has written about his experience on an elderly care ward:

■ *Staff nurse told me off this morning. I took too long taking Mr Brown to the toilet and he got upset – complained to staff nurse about me. I reckon she doesn't like male nurses.*

This bald statement of events is lacking in both detail and analysis. There is no reflection, no attempt to enquire into the reasons for Simon being told off, or for the patient becoming upset. Nothing is learned from these events and no plans are laid for preventing similar occurrences in the future. Instead, Simon tries to shift the responsibility for his telling off onto the staff nurse.

By contrast, this is what a more analytical Simon might have written. Notice how he has used headings as a means of structuring his log entry.

■ *What happened:*
  I feel bad today, not just because staff nurse told me off but because I upset Mr Brown. He'd asked me to help him to the toilet, and without thinking I replied, 'Yes, after I've finished taking these blood pressures'. By the time I got back to him he was sitting in a wet bed, crying.
■ *Points to learn:*
  a. I should have remembered that Mr Brown moves slowly, needs time to get to the toilet, and becomes very upset if he's incontinent.
  b. I should have organized my work into its proper priority – those blood pressures weren't urgent.
■ *To do:*
  a. Apologize properly to Mr Brown tomorrow.
  b. Keep a special eye on him and see to his needs quickly.
  c. Work out an order of priority for my jobs from now on.
  d. Choose the right moment to ask staff nurse if she will mention this incident on my ward report.

> The more reflective your learning log, the more useful it will be to your development. Use it not just to describe events, but to analyse them.

Here Simon has produced a more detailed, and far more useful, diary of events, with a plan of action attached. The following day's learning log will no doubt record how both the patient and the staff nurse responded to Simon's renewed efforts at delivering prioritized nursing care.

ACTIVITY

Can you improve on the second learning log? Are there other headings you can think of that might prompt Simon to think even more carefully and analytically about the events he's described? One heading might be 'My feelings', requiring him to consider what emotions he experienced after finding Mr Brown upset and incontinent. Such a heading could lead Simon to realize that not only did he experience shame and sorrow, but also disappointment at his own thoughtlessness, and embarrassment at meeting the patient again the next day.

Incidentally, Simon's supervisor would *not* allow this one unhappy event to influence the ward report she writes about him. Rather, she will observe how he responds to it. The second, more detailed diary excerpt seems to suggest that Simon has learned a great deal, and his nursing care will improve consequently.

Should a learning log be confidential? This question will probably be addressed by your college's assessment regulations which might, for instance, state that your ward supervisor should read your clinical learning log as part of your practical assessment. If this is the case, you should know about it *before* you begin writing your log. My preference would be for the log itself to remain confidential to the student who writes it, if she wishes. She may be asked to refer to it during her end of ward discussion with her tutor and supervisor, but the written pages themselves need not be handed over to her assessors.

WRITING FOR PUBLICATION

Keeping a daily diary is often practised by writers, not just as a record of events but as a review of moods and thoughts, and descriptions of people encountered, of scenes, sounds and smells. The difficulty is not so much starting a diary, as keeping it going.

One of the frustrations of writing is that ideas don't occur to you at the times you set aside for writing. You may plan to start writing at 9 a.m. on a Monday, but ideas ('inspiration' if you prefer) can't be booked to appear like a pantomime good fairy. There is nothing more daunting, nor more muse-destroying, than the conjunction of a blank sheet of paper and a ticking clock.

One of the *joys* of writing, by contrast, is that ideas will arrive unannounced and unsought, at odd times and in odder places. Such ideas will vanish from your mind as abruptly as they arrive, unless they are captured first on paper.

Forget personal organizers and word processors: a writer's greatest helpmate is a collection of small notebooks, each with its pen, scattered throughout his living quarters, including the kitchen, bathroom, and bedside table. Thoughts are jotted down as they arrive, and later transferred to a central store. There are two golden rules: never refrain from writing something down because you're too tired or busy. You'll be almost sure to forget it. And never remove any of the pens from their respective notebooks. Wherever there is a gap, an idea is sure to arrive.

Being assessed in your clinical placement

Planned effective learning will give rise to positive assessment results. By planning your clinical experience to address the learning outcomes laid down for you by your college curriculum, or negotiated individually with your tutor and supervisor, you stand a better chance of meeting those outcomes. Less useful is learning that is unplanned and haphazard, and a response to such 'accidental' learning that is uncritical and non-analytical. Clinical (or field) assessment and written assessment are two 'wings' of an overall assessment structure, and they are linked, not disparate. Each wing is as consciously planned as the other, and towards the end of this chapter I shall try and show how links can be forged between them, by both the curriculum planners and the student. Colleges plan their clinical assessment strategies just as they plan their clinical learning strategies. Clinical learning thus leads, logically and inevitably, to clinical assessment.

Your learning on a ward or in the community may well be guided by means of learning outcomes or objectives which you are required to meet. These are far more than lists of practical skills, such as recording a patient's temperature, collecting a sputum specimen, or showing a client how her stocking-aid works. For example, a student nurse may take a patient's temperature without understanding why she is doing so, or the significance of the raised temperature she finds. A student occupational therapist may demonstrate the use of a stocking-aid to a client without perceiving the role it plays in the client's determination to remain independent. Your learning outcomes, however, will set out appropriate skills for your level of training, and the knowledge and understanding underpinning those skills.

A third-year student nurse might have to meet learning outcomes such as these:

- The student will, under supervision, admit a non-emergency patient to the ward and carry out a preliminary nursing assessment, with reference to both the patient himself and, where applicable, any accompanying relatives.
- The student will make a verbal report to her supervisor concerning the patient she has admitted, including the reasons for his admission, his patient problems, and the possible nursing actions to help overcome those problems.
- The student will suggest how the care she proposes to deliver can be evaluated for its effectiveness.

The complexity of these learning outcomes is, I think, obvious. All three outcomes call for the student to use appropriate communication skills (towards the patient, relatives, and supervisor). They call for knowledge of normal and altered physiology, pharmacology (should the patient be taking medicines), psychology, and nursing theory and research. Such complex outcomes would be inappropriate for student nurses in the first year of training.

ACTIVITY

Study the learning outcomes or objectives established by your college curriculum. Find outcomes that have been designed for your first year practical placements, and compare them with related outcomes you must achieve in your third year. Discuss with colleagues how these outcomes differ, and how they are similar.

The practical learning outcomes or objectives that you face in successive years of study are tailored to fit the level of understanding deemed appropriate by your curriculum. You, too, play a part in tailoring these outcomes to suit your individual needs because you will decide, in consultation with your supervisor, *when* within a placement is the right time to be assessed. In short, you should aim to put yourself forward for assessment when you feel you will be successful. (This is particularly important if your contract of study allows you only a limited number of referrals.)

If you look at the order to events I set out earlier for the practice of giving injections, you can see how assessment comes towards the end of the process: not at the very end, because you never stop learning. (There will never come a point where you can

Practical assessments are best taken when you and your supervisor are certain you can pass them.

honestly tell yourself that you have nothing more to learn about a particular subject.) But the actual assessment is preceded by a long process of microskill practice, whole skill practice under supervision, going solo (but with the promise of help if required), and *then* the test. During this process, you will be assessing your own skills as well as receiving feedback from your supervisor.

Some notes on self-assessment

Self-assessment is a continuing process which begins, ideally, when you first set foot on your ward, or sally out into the community with your field leader. Self-assessment isn't, in my view, an optional extra, but a vital aspect of your personal and professional development. Forming the habit of assessing your own performance will stand you in good stead when, as a qualified practitioner, you no longer have the comfort of a supervisor close at hand. (As a new staff nurse, however, you should be working under the support and guidance of a mentor, an experienced and approachable senior nurse, for approximately the first year.)

It is through reflective practice that you self-assess, and you'll remember my earlier discussion about how maintaining a learning log can enhance the process of reflection. Simply muttering, 'I didn't do that dressing very well' as you clear away your trolley is an inadequate response to the inadequate care you feel you've delivered. 'Gut feelings' aren't reflective. It is by reflection that you face up to what factors made your work unsatisfactory. The headings and subheadings that you devise for your personal learning log will guide you towards a more organized session of reflection, and consequently a more satisfactory performance in the future.

This period of reflection need not be long. There will be times – at the end of a long and busy shift, for example – when you will feel too tired to bother about thinking through your day's performance. If you can combat such feelings, and reflect for just a few minutes in a methodical manner (guided by your learning log headings) you and your work will be the better for it.

It is good to receive positive feedback, however brief, from your supervisor – and the patient or client – at the end of your shift or when you finish a certain procedure. It is salutary to receive negative feedback too, provided it is delivered in a thoughtful and sensitive manner. But the advantage of getting into the habit of self-assessing is that you don't need the comments of others, though such comments can help to support the verdict you arrive at yourself.

I repeat the warning I gave earlier: don't be afraid to *praise* yourself. Don't indulge in a modesty trip which turns out to be, frankly, dishonest. If you did perform well, it is simply untrue to say that you didn't. A related warning might also be given here: don't be afraid to receive praise from others, including your client and supervisor. You might feel embarrassed if you're told that you performed really well in a difficult situation, but don't dismiss such feedback. Utter a grateful 'thank you' and store the praise away in your memory banks ready for future, rockier periods in your career. You are almost certain to need it.

Some notes on assessment by others

The purpose of clinical or field supervision is to guide you towards assessment with a positive outcome. Learning objectives you are required to meet on a surgical ward, or intensive care unit, or in a day hostel, *must* be met in order that you pass the assessment.

Just as I advised, in earlier chapters, that you gain a clear understanding of your college regulations concerning written assessment, so I strongly suggest that you

On any practical placement, find out **who** is to assess you, **when**, and on what skills.

make yourself familiar with the clinical outcomes or objectives, including those 'core' outcomes which must be passed, for each placement.

You should be clear about **who** is going to assess you (your supervisor, another clinician, or a tutor from college); clear about **when** you are going to be assessed (during every shift, or towards the end of the placement); and clear about **what** is going to be assessed.

You may, for example, be a second-year student nurse who is allocated to a surgical ward. You work for one or two shifts each week with your named supervisor or her deputy. This week you are caring for the postoperative patients in one bay of the ward. Celia, your supervisor, tells you that you are making good progress. 'How do you feel about being assessed by Robert and me on Friday?'

You may initially be thrown by this question – the actual moment of assessment is looming all too close! But wait a minute – you've helped your supervisor to collect patients from the recovery room of the theatre block; you've given many of your patients painkilling injections, and you know about the regulations concerning controlled drugs such as morphine; and you've taken out a whole row of clips from someone's abdomen. You've cared for patients who feel sick after a general anaesthetic, and you've measured output from urinary catheters and wound drains. You've sat with a very ill patient after a long operation and taken his pulse and blood pressure every 15 minutes.

All of this you have done and, according to your supervisor and her deputy, done well. You really are ready for the assessment. It is important that your assessment concentrates on the practical skills and knowledge you have gained in the previous few weeks. For example, if during your assessment a patient with a heart monitor is admitted to your bay, and you have never nursed someone with one of these machines, it would be unfair to penalize you because you don't know what the various heart rhythms mean.

However, it *would* be fair to assess your reaction to something that happens unexpectedly, such as a fire alarm sounding, or one of your patients suffering a cardiac arrest. I would expect a second-year student nurse to be able to diagnose a cardiac arrest, call for the 'crash' team, and begin resuscitation. (I would expect *any* health care student and professional to be capable of this.) You cannot claim that such an event is unfair during your assessment, because nothing of the sort happened in the preceding few weeks on the ward.

You will have noticed in the above brief scenario that you were to be assessed by both your supervisor and her deputy. Usually, towards the end of a clinical placement, the decision to pass or refer will be taken by a small group of qualified practitioners, including the ward manager. No one person will, alone, have the responsibility of referring you. This reduces the risk of personality clashes unduly influencing your assessment.

Any problems that emerge during the placement will be discussed with your personal tutor, *and with you*. A referral on a clinical placement should never come as a surprise. This is why it is usual for students to discuss their progress at an intermediate stage of the placement with their supervisors. It is unacceptable for a student to wait until the very end of his ward placement to be told that he is unsafe. If qualified nurses or therapists feel that a student is unsafe carrying out care, or his communication skills are poor, they *must* discuss the problem with him when it is first noticed.

During such a discussion, both supervisor and student (and perhaps the personal tutor too) will agree certain goals to be achieved during the remainder of the placement. The purpose of establishing these goals is to give the student something to work towards, week by week, so that she can eventually pass the clinical placement as a whole.

Here is an example similar to one used earlier. Susan, a third-year student nurse, is interviewed by her supervisor and the ward manager during the middle of her placement on a surgical ward. During the interview she is told that her knowledge of drugs appears to be poor. 'When you helped me with the medicine round this morning,' observes her supervisor, 'you knew hardly any of the drugs we gave to our patients, let alone their side effects. This means you wouldn't know what observations to make on your patients.'

Susan is asked to comment on this, or to challenge it. She may feel, for example, that she is at too junior a stage in her training to know much about the drugs used on the ward. The ward manager will doubtless robustly disagree. The matter is not left there, but together they discuss what each of them can do to overcome the problem. In other words, the interview doesn't remain negative; it ends on a positive note, with all parties agreeing (perhaps contracting) to carry out certain actions. Susan might contract to learn:

- 6 analgesics commonly used on the ward
- 6 antibiotics commonly used on the ward
- 3 intravenous infusion fluids commonly used on the ward

making detailed notes on each, which she will show to her supervisor. The latter contracts to test Susan on her newly gained knowledge, and to take her on three more medicine rounds on the ward. The ward manager contracts to take Susan on a medicine round towards the end of her placement.

The outcome of the intermediate interview is that Susan, made aware of deficiencies in her knowledge, is encouraged to set about improving matters. Out of that negative criticism, something positive emerges.

It is important to state here that you should not be referred on a clinical placement on the basis of one error or misjudgement. Where an unfortunate incident occurs, such as a student letting a 'drip' run through too quickly, the matter is dealt with *at the time*. The occurrence is examined and discussed, and plans made to see that it doesn't happen again. Then the matter is closed. Nothing is served, I would suggest, by dragging up incidents which by then have whiskers on them at the final interview of a clinical placement. By then, any necessary learning change will have occurred, or not. The final interview is simply too late.

Where, however, intermediate interviews with a student produce no change in knowledge, skill, or attitude, and where no improvement in performance is noticed, supervisors and ward managers have the right to consider awarding a refer (or fail) grade at the final interview. In my experience as a nurse tutor, I have observed how very reluctant ward nurses and managers are to fail a student. This is not in the least because they have low standards or expectations but, I think, because they understand the implications of failing a student. You may remember that I made a similar comment about the attitude of teachers marking written examinations, and how reluctant they are to fail a student, especially when it is a final examination.

Sometimes a ward manager has asked me, as the ward tutor, for guidance about a student who appears to be heading towards a referral. The first thing I make clear to the manager and the student's supervisor is that the final decision is theirs. I will not dictate, nor will I challenge, any decision they make. Then I ask them to summarize what progress they feel the student has made on their ward:

- What knowledge and skills did the student bring to the ward at the beginning of her placement?
- What knowledge and skills will the student take with her when she leaves the ward?
- Therefore, what learning has occurred on the ward, and what changes can be perceived in the student's attitudes, skills, and behaviour?

Each student comes to the clinical or field placement, even the very first, with her personal 'baggage', in the form of life experience, specific knowledge, practical skills, and attitudes towards people and events. One of the functions of a preliminary student interview is to make a record of this 'baggage'. Any deficit in knowledge and skills is also recorded, and ways devised to make good such deficit. Throughout the placement, but particularly at the intermediate and final interviews, the student's progress will be observed and her baggage examined for gain or loss.

This, I think, is the key question concerning whether a student passes or fails a practical placement: has any significant learning occurred? At the end of 10 weeks on a paediatric ward, for example, Bill may admit to his supervisor that he is more convinced than ever that paediatric nursing is not for him. This will not earn him an automatic fail! He may also say that he has been impressed by how the ward seeks to involve parents in the care of their children. He adds, 'I've learned more about communication skills here than on any of the adult wards I've been so far.'

By careful questioning, the supervisor seeks examples of such skills, in order to ensure that Bill is aware of the scope of his newly gained knowledge. At the end of the interview she is happy to tell Bill that he has passed his unloved yet valuable paediatric experience.

The assessment process again – how practical and theoretical assessments are linked

This book began with a discussion of the overall assessment process in health care courses. In that discussion, I demonstrated how the various tests (essays, care studies, or exams) heading towards the student fitted into a logical process. Have another look at Figure 1.1 just to refresh your memory, and perhaps read the first chapter again.

In these next few paragraphs I want to show how both written and practical assessments similarly fit into one assessment process. I hesitate to use the phrase 'theoretical assessment' for the former, because that might seem to suggest that practical work and practical assessment have no theoretical input. Nevertheless, it seems to be the experience of some students that they have difficulty in perceiving how their classroom learning links with their learning on the wards and in the community. It is, of course, up to teachers to promote the perception of such links, as well as for students to seek them out for themselves.

Figure 12.2 shows how links can be formed between classroom and ward or community learning. The subject matter is familiar, in that I've used it before: a patient or client with rheumatoid arthritis. This subject may present itself in the form of a client you visit in her own home, or a patient admitted to a hospital ward for assessment. It may present itself in the form of an essay or exam question: 'Discuss the effects of rheumatoid arthritis on the individual's ability to care for herself'. (I have chosen this subject because I think it is relevant to physiotherapists, occupational therapists, and nurses.)

The diagram shows how new knowledge builds on what has been formerly gained, both in classroom learning and practical experience. You start, at the bottom of the figure, with the normal anatomy and physiology of certain joints (such as the hand), something that is learned from textbooks, and which can be observed in patients and clients with normal joint movement. You then have the chance to observe a client with badly deformed hands where the arthritic condition has attacked the various joints, and to note how the client struggles to lift a cup to her mouth. The knowledge base which assists your observation is derived from your classroom learning of the pathology of rheumatoid arthritis, and your textbooks and lectures, perhaps enhanced by examining X-rays of diseased joints. Book learning and classroom learning don't have to precede practical placement learning. It can occur

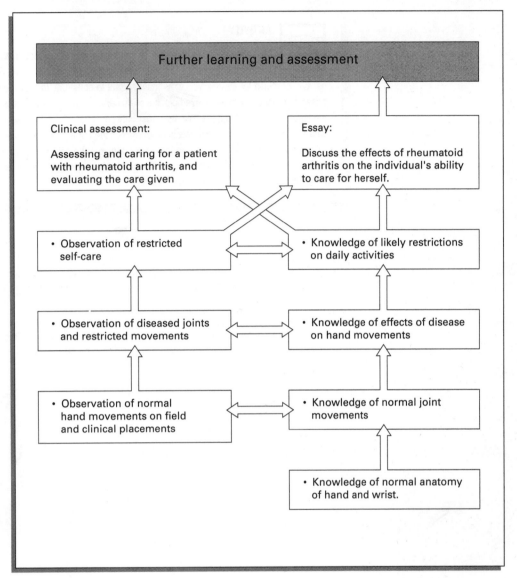

Further learning and assessment

Clinical assessment:

Assessing and caring for a patient with rheumatoid arthritis, and evaluating the care given

Essay:

Discuss the effects of rheumatoid arthritis on the individual's ability to care for herself.

• Observation of restricted self-care

• Knowledge of likely restrictions on daily activities

• Observation of diseased joints and restricted movements

• Knowledge of effects of disease on hand movements

• Observation of normal hand movements on field and clinical placements

• Knowledge of normal joint movements

• Knowledge of normal anatomy of hand and wrist.

Figure 12.2
How written and practical assessments occur within the learning and assessment processes. These assessments lead to further learning experiences and assessment possibilities.

the other way round, with your observation of a newly admitted patient sending you, full of curiosity, to your books when you get off duty. In your books you find the explanation for those swollen joints that look so hot and painful.

When you come to write your exam answer, your past experience of assisting a client with rheumatoid arthritis helps you to formulate a well planned and detailed essay. Your knowledge of the client's problems with various daily activities will come not only from books and lectures, but also from your observation on the wards or in the client's own home.

Similarly, when you are assessed on your practical care of the client, your knowledge and skills demonstrated during that care are not simply gained from your preceding practical experience. Classroom learning is incorporated here too. You understand the client's problems in handling a drinking cup, because you understand what has happened to her hand joints.

ACTIVITY

I have always found it helpful, when teaching, to recall patients that I have actually nursed, and students writing exam answers tell me this is beneficial for them, too. When you come to plan essays, or revise for exams, you may find it helpful to construct your own diagrams, similar to Figure 12.2, based on other conditions (for example, the client suffering from a heart attack, or the child with asthma). Such a diagram clearly sets out the links that exist between what you've learned in the classroom and library, and what you've gained from your practical experience. If there are gaps in your own diagrams, these may point you to areas where you need to concentrate your learning – the pathophysiology of asthma, for example, or the convalescent care of a heart attack client. The point about constructing such diagrams is that they will accurately reflect the state of your own learning.

REFERENCES

Anforth P 1992 Mentors, not assessors. Nurse Education Today 12: 299–302

Armitage P, Burnard P 1991 Mentors or preceptors: narrowing the theory-practice gap. Nurse Education Today 11: 225–229

Barlow S 1991 Impossible dream. Nursing Times 87 (1): 53–54

ENB Circular 39/APS. English National Board, London

Goodall C 1985 A student tutor's evaluation of his teaching placement. Nurse Education Today 5: 95–100

Morris N, John G, Keen T 1988 Learning the ropes. Nursing Times 84 (46): 24–27

Morton-Cooper A, Palmer A 1993 Mentoring and preceptorship: a guide to support roles in clinical practice. Blackwell Scientific Publications, Oxford

Postscript: Dealing with failure

Wherever summative assessment exists, by definition there also exists the possibility of failing. It is likely that readers of this book will, through their own efforts and those of their tutors and supervisors, satisfactorily complete all their assessments and take their places as qualified health care professionals. For others, the outcome may not be so happy.

Different colleges and different courses have varying pass rates, and you may find this information in the college handbook sent out to you as a prospective applicant seeking information about where to apply for your health care course. If not, you could justifiably ask about it during an informal visit or interview. (Remember that interviews are for you to ask questions, as much as to answer them.)

Be careful how you use such information, though. Don't assume that a college with a 90% pass rate is somehow 'better' than one with a 70% rate. Neither should you assume that the latter has a stricter assessment strategy than the former. Make sure, also, that the percentage you are given is an average for, say, 2 or 3 years, and not a particularly favourable single example. Nevertheless, there is some comfort to be gained from being in an educational situation with a consistently high pass rate. This might suggest, for example, that students are assessed at that point in their courses where they are very likely to pass.

Failures occur, however, and the important question concerns how you face up to failing or being referred should it happen to you. The following remarks concern referral in an assessment where a retake is allowed – in other words, an assessment which is partly formative. You may have to resubmit a care study, or resit an exam, or undergo a particular practical placement again. What is important for all these is the way in which you approach your referral.

The worst thing to do, when failure occurs, is to seek to pin the blame squarely on other people or other things, anything but yourself: the exam room was too hot and the invigilator's shoes squeaked; the essay questions were especially hard or in some way 'unfair'; your teachers gave you wrong advice about revising; your teachers' lectures were wrong; you had a cold or hay fever. The list is endless, yet it is one with which, I guess, many tutors will be familiar. How refreshing it is to meet a student who admits: yes, I didn't revise hard enough, I didn't organize my time sufficiently, and I misread the first question I attempted.

Facing up to *your* responsibility for your referral is the first major step in retaking the assessment . . . and passing.

Wait for a little while, after receiving the bad news, for your natural disappointment (and perhaps even your anger) to quieten. It is perfectly natural to feel rotten after learning that you've failed an exam or had an essay referred. Those first few hours or days are not the best time for seeking constructive advice, yet this is what you must eventually do.

Please remember that your referred exam or essay will have been marked by at least two experienced markers, who will have tried hard to pass you. When you feel you've recovered a little of your poise, perhaps when you feel a little less angry with yourself, go to your tutor and seek her advice. It is your right to receive detailed, accurate advice. It is perfectly possible for teachers to provide such guidance even when they have to protect the identity of the markers.

Comments such as, 'You needed a bit more detail in places', are simply not good enough. It is the mark of an educationally sound institution that its teachers can evaluate students' work in sufficient detail as to be of some practical value – which isn't, I think, too much to ask.

Here is the sort of detailed advice you should receive (concerning an imaginary failed essay):

■ *The main problem seemed to lie in the apparent lack of planning. Your introduction was too short and failed to set out what you wanted your essay to show. The discussion that followed dealt with three important areas of the subject matter, but the links between these areas simply weren't made. Consequently, your essay appeared to be very disjointed, and I lost any sense of a developing argument. You omitted any mention of subjects X and Y; perhaps your introduction could have explained that you intended to do this, leaving your argument based on the three factors you actually chose. 'I'm going to discuss A, B and C, but lack of time means I shall have to leave aside X and Y' – something like that. Finally, there was no effective conclusion in which to draw together your arguments. I got the impression that you ran out of either time or interest in the subject.*

As to the essay's content, you included an adequate number of references, though they were all rather 'elderly'. You missed out, however, any mention of your own clinical experience, so that this essay might have been written by a student not on a health care course.

How does this sound to you? By discussing such comments with you, your tutor can lead you towards a rewriting of your essay with especial concentration on its overall planning. Such advice should act as a *guide*. You should come away from your tutorial knowing clearly what measures to adopt for a successful retake.

Your role is to examine carefully the comments you receive, and to engage with them in order to accept your own role in putting matters right. It is terribly sad, in my experience, to see a student unwilling even to engage with the advice that is offered, let alone accept it. She looks for any and every scapegoat for her referral, and so misses the true cause as well as any opportunity to put matters right. You cannot improve something which you don't accept needs improving.

But that is too unhappy a manner in which to end this book, which is meant to be positive and encouraging – a desktop friend for you. It is my experience that the majority of students readily accept their responsibility in any referrals that occur. Indeed, it is sometimes the case that their self-criticism is far more negative than the comments provided by the teachers. So I shall end by repeating the advice I've given before more than once: don't hesitate to admit your successes, your good points, and your achievements. To 'criticize' is not to be destructive. You really are allowed both to praise yourself whenever you think it is appropriate, and to accept praise from others.

Notes

N o t e s

Index